LEADERSHIP FOR

SMOOTH PATIENT

FLOW

Improved Outcomes

Improved Service

Improved Bottom Line

LEADERSHIP FOR SMOOTH PATIENT FLOW

Improved Outcomes
Improved Service
Improved Bottom Line

Kirk Jensen

Thom A. Mayer

Shari J. Welch

Carol Haraden

ACHE Management Series

Health Administration Press

Your board, staff, or clients may also benefit from this book's insight. For more information on quantity discounts, contact the Health Administration Press Marketing Manager at (312) 424-9470.

11   10   09   08   5   4   3   2

Library of Congress Cataloging-in-Publication Data

Leadership for smooth patient flow : improved outcomes, improved service, improved bottom line / Kirk Jensen... [et al.].
      p. cm.
Includes bibliographical references.
ISBN-13: 978-1-56793-265-2
ISBN-10: 1-56793-265-7 (alk. paper)
1. Hospitals—Administration. 2. Hospitals—Admission and discharge. I. Jensen, Kirk, 1952-
RA971.8.L385 2006
362.11068—dc22

                                                        2006049608

Acquisitions editor: Audrey Kaufman; Project manager: Gregory Sebben; Layout editor: Chris Underdown; Cover designer: Trisha Lartz

Health Administration Press
A division of the Foundation of the
   American College of Healthcare Executives
1 North Franklin Street, Suite 1700
Chicago, IL 60606-3424
(312) 424-2800

Contents

To my best friend and terrific wife, Karen, who has been there with me every step of the way, and to our sons Christopher and Michael, for their joy, humor, and inquisitiveness. I appreciate their patience and sacrifice as I have pursued this passion. And to my parents, Earl and Naomi Jensen, who were there at the beginning

— *Kirk Jensen*

To my beautiful and brilliant wife, Maureen, and our kind, generous, and thoughtful sons Josh, Kevin, and Gregory. They exhibited uncommon patience with the hard work, long hours, and travel to every corner of the country that were necessary to complete our research on patient flow. Their love and support have sustained me in this and all other work.

— *Thom A. Mayer*

To Sam and Emma, for eating pot pies so their mother could finish these chapters.

— *Shari J. Welch*

To my son Jacob, whose humor and fun-loving spirit help keep life and work in perspective.

— *Carol Haraden*

Acknowledgments

WE WOULD LIKE to acknowledge first and foremost our fellow authors in this endeavor, whose wisdom, foresight, and dedication to improving patient flow are truly exemplary. Our friends and colleagues at BestPractices, Inc., with whom we have the opportunity to work every day, are as fine a team of healthcare leaders as any in the nation, and their thoughts have contributed greatly to our understanding of patient flow. These individuals include Raul Armengol, Damian Banaszak, Glenn Druckenbrod, Bob Cates, Luis Eljaiek Jr., Dan Hanfling, John Howell, Peter Paganussi, Denis Pauze, Rick Place, Ben Winter, Anthony Kitchen, Wayne Cayton, Jim Klein, Saeed Rehman, Jeff Berry, Michael Boyle, Gary Senula, and Michal Born. We would also like to thank our friends and colleagues at the Institute for Healthcare Improvement, in particular, Don Berwick, Roger Resar, Eugene Litvak, Diane Jacobsen, and Marilyn Rudolph.

Joy Sparks-Gaviria was, as always, a "joy to work with" and her painstaking attention to detail in the creation of portions of the manuscript are greatly appreciated. Thanks also to Sabrina Hunt, who cheerfully and thoughtfully helped to assemble and dispatch many pieces of traveling manuscript.

We would like to express our sincerest gratitude to Daphne O'Brien for her hard work and commitment in her contributions. Her insight, gift with language, and incredible sense of humor were invaluable.

We would also like to thank Audrey Kaufman at Health Administration Press who was, in many ways, as much a creator and guiding force to this work as the authors themselves. No authors could ever have better leadership from their editor than Audrey has provided.

I (Kirk) owe deep gratitude to my friends and mentors at Associates in Process Improvement, Kevin Nolan and Tom Nolan, and to the faculty and my colleagues at the University of Tennessee Physician MBA Program. Their help and support have been invaluable.

And finally, thanks to the patients and healthcare institutions who have allowed us to both learn and practice the art and science of medicine and healthcare system operations. If we have neglected to mention any of the many others who have contributed to our lives and our thinking about patient flow, it is simply because of space limitations and does not reflect the depth of our gratitude and appreciation.

Foreword

THE QUALITY IMPROVEMENT movement in American healthcare reached a distinct turning point in December of 1999 with the publication of the landmark report on patient safety, *To Err Is Human*, by the Institute of Medicine (IOM). For decades, students of healthcare quality carefully documented defects in care—many of them egregious—with little reaction from either the public or the professions. A gap existed, not just between the performance and the scientific potential of healthcare (a gap that the subsequent IOM report on quality would call "a chasm"), but also between beliefs and facts about just how good, or bad, was American healthcare.

To Err Is Human took an enormous step toward closing the latter gap. In temperate language, based soundly in evidence, the IOM report clearly informed our nation that healthcare was fundamentally unsafe, that tens of thousands of Americans died each year from avoidable errors in healthcare rather than from their diseases, and that modern scientific approaches to safety held great potential for productive redesigns with much lower inherent hazards. Within days of publication, the IOM report was front-page news in both professional and lay media. Those of us involved in crafting the report found ourselves in a maelstrom of interviews in television, radio, and print publications. And the storm continued for weeks, even months, afterward. Even now, seven years after the report appeared, reporters call me almost every week to explore and track the healthcare safety story.

Someone not involved professionally in the study of healthcare quality may have difficulty understanding how fundamental a change this was. Year after year, I joined many scientific colleagues in trying to gain the attention of leaders who might, if they had the will, improve healthcare greatly. Year after year, we tried to alert the public to the facts about how much better their care could be with proper changes in processes and designs. But the response was small, muted, and evanescent. Until, that is, *To Err Is Human* appeared. Since that day, we have had the attention of both leaders and the public.

Why? Why did patient safety emerge so dramatically as the breakthrough issue in awareness and concern about the quality of care? The answer, I think, has something to do with a convergence of properties of the safety problem: it is charismatic (people can grasp it and care about it), it is big (with echoes in the direct experiences of patients, finances, and disease burden), it is pervasive (affecting almost every corner of care), it is interesting (with technical dimensions that almost anyone with time to study the matter will find novel and intellectually stimulating), and it is remediable (with sound theory guiding bold action).

So, patient safety became, and remains, the leading-edge problem in the field of healthcare quality. With the second IOM report, *Crossing the Quality Chasm*, released in 2001, safety joined five siblings—effectiveness, patient centeredness, timeliness, efficiency, and equity—as "aims for improvement of healthcare," but safety is without much doubt the most charismatic among those aims.

Not long after safety leapt to the top, I became aware of a second "sleeping giant" of a problem in care—"flow." It was my close colleague and mentor, Tom Nolan, who first gave it a name for me. He asserted that "flow through the system" was an issue in some ways every bit as crucial and challenging as "safety," and that, like safety, the issue of flow had somehow become cut off in healthcare from the foundational sciences that, correctly employed, could help break healthcare free of some costly fetters. The problem of flow in healthcare may not have the charisma of safety, but it has everything else: it is big (indeed, gigantic!), pervasive, interesting, and highly remediable.

With Tom Nolan's guidance, the Institute for Healthcare Improvement (IHI) soon initiated a family of efforts to bring systems sciences to the problems of flow in healthcare. The problems loomed larger and larger as we became more familiar with them and, equally, the complexity and promise of the relevant scientific viewpoints on flow became ever more impressive. Though "flow" lacked the charisma of "safety" for many professionals and almost all laypeople, we found resonance immediately in the minds and will of the vast majority of healthcare managers and executives, whose day-to-day work reminded them continually of the costs and burdens associated with interruptions in continuous flow throughout their organizations—patients awaiting admission, patients awaiting discharge, queues for tests and procedures, pervasive cancellations, emergency room diversions, crowded waiting rooms, idle and frustrated clinicians, empty operating theaters adjacent to overbooked operating theaters—the symptoms went on and on.

A faculty formed in IHI that was deeply devoted to the study of flow and approaches to its improvement, and the authors of *Leadership for Smooth Patient Flow* emerged as senior among the group. As in the world of patient safety, the intellectual challenges in the sciences of flow proved to be of two major types—to master the complex theories and approaches that had matured in other industries and academic disciplines far from healthcare, and, at the same time, to adapt and invent new theories helpful in the special contexts of healthcare systems. Scholars such as IHI senior fellows Eugene Litvak and Steven Spear helped us in both endeavors, and skills and insights grew. We learned a ton.

Leadership for Smooth Patient Flow marks a milestone in the ability to explain and explore flow as a central, improvable property of healthcare systems. It will help any leader who both respects and cares about this problem and who is willing to tackle the fascinating combination of technical and sociological challenges that improving flow encounters. The authors are masters of both theory and application, and they speak from real experiences bravely met.

Will flow ever acquire the patina of charisma that fuels today's work on patient safety? I doubt it. Flow is one step too complex, and one step too far removed from daily language. But, whether so honored or not, the problem of flow is every bit as consequential for the health of our systems and the well-being of our patients. Properly addressed, the improvement of flow will yield dividends for every dimension of quality of care—safety included—and, in that sense, it may turn out, on reflection, to be not the poor younger sibling of safety, but its elder.

—Donald M. Berwick, M.D.
President and CEO
Institute for Healthcare Improvement

References

Institute of Medicine. 1999. *To Err Is Human: Building a Safer Health System*. Washington, D.C.: National Academies Press.

————.2001. *Crossing the Quality Chasm: A New Health System for the 21st Century*. Washington, D.C.: National Academies Press.

Preface

WATCHING AN EXPERT skier glide down a difficult run, we see a linked progression of turns that, taken as a whole, is a thing of beauty. John Musser (2002) of Alta, Utah, who is consistently rated as one of North America's top ski instructors, put it this way:

> Expert skiers flow down the mountain like water, taking the path where gravity takes them. It is not a straight line, but a logical path, linking one turn with the next, as gravity pulls them down the mountain.

When smooth flow is experienced in the healthcare system, whether from the perspective of the patient or the provider, it seems that the care provided has a logical, nearly inexorable progression, where the elements of care are linked together, one after another.

Yet much of our healthcare system doesn't "follow gravity"—indeed, it often seems to *defy* gravity. We so often find ourselves working in systems where we are always trying to push rather than pull—push patients through to the examining room, push emergency department admits into the cardiac unit, and push discharges through the business office. Many healthcare organizations have recognized that the transfer of patients from one unit to another should be subject to a pull system, rather than a push system. It makes more sense that receiving units should be actively pulling patients from the transferring units, rather than having to rely on the transferring unit to push the patient toward them. It is a simple matter of energy transfer—as it were, following the laws of gravity.

In healthcare, it would serve us well if we spent less time thinking, "What's the policy, what's the procedure?," and more time thinking, "What's the next logical step for this patient?" In other words, where does the gravity of patient care take us?

From the patient's perspective, flow occurs when studies or procedures are followed promptly by results—simple answers to simple questions. Recently, while covering a lacrosse game as a team physician, one of us was approached by a parent of one of the players, who related his story this way:

> **"Doc, I could really use your help."**

> "What can I do to help you?"

> **"I had a cardiac CT, which showed a high calcium score, and my doctor had me get an immediate stress-thallium test."**

> "So your stress test shows significant cardiac disease? Because I can recommend a great team of cardiologists and cardiovascular surgeons for you!"

> **"No, that isn't it."**

> "So what's the problem?"

> **"I haven't gotten any results—and it's been five days."**

Can you imagine having no test results after five days? Would you tolerate that? A five-day delay after being told an immediate stress test was needed! And yet it happens every day in our healthcare system. If the poor guy did have cardiac disease, it's a miracle he didn't have a myocardial infarction from the stress of waiting! In fact, the wait for the results was probably more of a stress test than the procedure itself. Like gravity, it seems simple that results should flow back to the patient as a logical next step, particularly when we are talking about something as serious as cardiac disease.

In this book, we offer our perspectives on making the shift from push to pull in your own healthcare system—on improving patient flow. While we do not always describe the innovations under discussion in terms of "push" or "pull," this gravity is the context in which we explore changes that have helped healthcare organizations all over the world improve the healthcare experience for their patients and providers. We know these strategies work: we have used them ourselves and we have helped others to use them.

We begin with a definition of flow that stretches beyond the commonplace. Chapter 1 examines the meaning of flow through five lenses, concluding with a patient flow matrix perspective that synthesizes the others. Flow is defined as much more than turnaround time or length of stay, encompassing such areas as systems thinking, reduced variability, and meeting and exceeding expectations.

After exploring the meaning of flow, we look in Chapter 2 at the specific benefits of undertaking improvements in flow for the patient, the healthcare team, and administration. In other words, we answer the question, "Why go to the trouble of making changes to improve flow? What's the advantage?" In this section we examine the relationship between flow and patient safety and satisfaction. We also look at how healthcare providers benefit from good flow and at the administrative and regulatory issues that make flow improvement a not-to-be-missed opportunity. Because change should be justified by the bottom line, we devote an entire chapter to exploring the business rationale for improving flow.

Chapter 3 makes the business case, showing the connection between increased profitability and the benefits for patients, the healthcare team, and administration. In this chapter, we look at both the "hard green dollars" and "soft green dollars" that come with improved flow.

With all the benefits explored and the bottom-line advantage established, we take a look in Chapter 4 at the leadership challenges inherent in leading change and suggest strategies on which to build to achieve leadership in patient flow. We establish flow improvement as a worthwhile but complex technical challenge that demands an understanding of human nature and an ability to subsume personal goals to those of the system as a whole. Change leadership is about teamwork.

Chapter 5 explores service industry theories and principles that are adaptable to healthcare systems. What does Disney know about keeping customers happy that you can use to improve your patients' experiences in your hospital? What can we learn from the Ritz-Carlton ("ladies and gentlemen serving ladies and gentlemen")? What do McDonald's and Starbucks know about demand-capacity planning or preparing for unscheduled demand that we can adapt to our own workplaces? We'll tell you. We also explore the metrics that determine how well these principles are working when they are applied to healthcare flow. We look at benchmarking and optimum turnaround times for segments of the service cycle to give you a way to evaluate your system and to set goals.

Chapter 6 is a primer for looking at your systems, focusing on making the emergency department and the rest of the system work together, pulling patients through in a caring, considerate, planned, inclusive, and progressive way. This chapter includes a toolkit of strategies that have worked the best for us and others in our flow improvement efforts.

What we offer here is a compendium of our collective experiences—what we have learned from our successes and our failures. Healthcare improvement—smoothing the flow—is a journey rather than a destination. It is a quest to improve the quality of life for you and for the patients you serve. To borrow and tweak a phrase from Norman McLean, "A river runs through us," made up of patients who come to us to heal and to be cared for. This river flows through our communities and through our healthcare organizations. It is meaningful work that we do. We offer these experiences to help you make that work easier and more satisfying for you and your patients. Let the journey begin!

References

Musser, J. 2002. Personal communication with Thom Mayer, March 24.

CHAPTER 1

Defining Flow

OUR FIRST TASK in improving flow is to define it. As healthcare leaders, we want precision and focus in our vision of flow, particularly since we must communicate that vision to others in an actionable way. One way to come to a practical definition of flow is by looking at it from a series of different perspectives—through a series of different "lenses" that allow us to see flow with more acuity. Just as an ophthalmologist has a patient look through a series of lenses as she finds the proper refraction, the process of using "lenses" to view flow should allow us to see it more clearly.

What follows in this chapter is a series of "lenses" through which we will look at flow to lead us to a pragmatic definition, applicable to any initiative designed to improve flow. Any serious, practical definition of a complex concept such as patient flow in healthcare must always involve elements of seeming incongruity that ultimately come together as a meaningful whole. Or, as the great physicist Niels Bohr once said, "The opposite of a correct statement is a false statement. The opposite of a profound truth may be another profound truth."

With that wisdom in mind, let us explore the definition of flow. As we begin, one caveat is necessary. Flow, while looked at globally by healthcare leaders, is always about our patients—it is the journey of our patients through our healthcare system in a way that encompasses the five features that follow.

1. FLOW AS EFFICIENCY AND CYCLE TIMES

The simplest way to view patient flow is as the outcome of an efficient or timely healthcare process. Taken to its lowest common denominator, is flow simply turnaround time (TAT)? Certainly, TAT is an extremely important part of the patient experience. Basic healthcare economics predicts that effectively reducing cost while producing the fastest feasible TATs results in faster "bed turns," which results in improved profitability. In the emergency department (ED), most patients perceive that "fast is good." A variety of patients with multiple levels of acuity are seen in the ED at any given time, on any given day. Creating a "Fast Track" area in the ED to treat minor illnesses and injuries is an example of creating efficiency and improved TAT for a specific group or segment of patients, thereby improving patient flow. Sprained ankles, minor infectious diseases, and minor trauma can all be taken care of in such units where the primary metric is TAT (since quality in treating minor problems is often assumed). For these patients with minor illnesses or injuries, flow and TAT may be nearly synonymous. Nonetheless, in an environment of fixed ED resources, does increasing flow for Fast Track patients off load demand and smooth flow for other ED patients? It certainly can, depending on the design and implementation of the Fast Track program and whether resources are added to create the program or merely diverted from other areas. Appropriately segmenting and optimizing patient flow for groups of patients can be a powerful patient flow tool when used appropriately.

Expanding on the ED example, the single most common complaint seen in most EDs is nonspecific abdominal pain. While the goal is to see these patients in a timely and efficient fashion, the clinical evaluation and treatment of abdominal pain (as well as many other patient complaints) takes time, including the time to evaluate the patient's response to therapy. Imaging studies and appropriate diagnostic tests also take time, all of which we want to hold to a minimum, but which, taken as a whole, mean that we are not likely to be able to see patients with nonspecific abdominal pain as quickly as we see Fast Track patients. Thus, in most EDs, turnaround time alone is an inadequate metric to assess flow. Be mindful of the difference between value-added and non–value-added process time. In emergency medicine, as well as in many other areas in the hospital, we should be "fast at fast things, and slow at slow things." The difficulty arises when we use strictly time-related metrics for issues that have a more complex and more contextual process associated with them.

> It's not just how much time you spend; it's how you spend the time.
> —Thom A. Mayer

Efficiency, effectiveness and turnaround time are extremely important elements of the flow definition, but they are inadequate in completely addressing the complex concept of flow.

2. FLOW AS REDUCED VARIATION, INCREASED PREDICTABILITY, AND IMPROVED FORECASTING

The Institute for Healthcare Improvement (IHI) has been a leader in improving the quality of healthcare for several decades. Under the leadership of a visionary Chief Executive Officer (CEO), Dr. Donald Berwick, IHI has convened a series of "collaboratives" and innovation teams, and has been at the forefront of addressing the issue of patient flow. IHI's white paper monograph titled *Optimizing Patient Flow: Moving Patients Smoothly Through Acute Care Settings* (IHI 2003) presents the following definition of flow: "IHI believes the key to improving flow lies in reducing process variation that impacts flow."

This definition extends beyond simply looking at efficiency or turnaround time and focuses on the extremely important issue of unnecessary variation as a key culprit in causing dysfunctional flow. A series of tools and techniques have been developed by IHI and others to help eliminate bottlenecks and unnecessary delays, primarily through statistical analysis of variation in healthcare processes and reduction or even elimination of this variation, thereby improving the patient flow through the system.

With reduction of variation as a core component of the definition of flow, several important principles apply. First, all processes are subject to natural variation, which refers to variation that occurs due to the randomness of the disease process in and of itself. The innovative flow researcher Eugene Litvak (Litvak, Buerhaus, and Davidoff 2005) astutely makes the point that only under the following three conditions could variation in healthcare be eliminated:

1. All patients would have to have the same disease, with the same severity.
2. All patients would have to arrive at the same time and/or rate per hour.
3. All providers would have to be equal, not just in their ability to care for the disease, but in the actual implementation of that ability with patients.

Litvak and colleagues further note that these conditions are never attained in healthcare, nor could they possibly be, which means that inherent and natural variation is unavoidable. Carol Haraden and Roger Resar (2004) point out in their study of patient flow that natural variation is present everywhere in healthcare, but also that it plays a far less important role than many believe, since natural variation "can affect flow, but commonly plays a small role and tends to be relatively constant in the system."

In contradistinction to natural variation, artificial variation in healthcare occurs because of personal preferences or differences in ability to care for the patient with a given disease. Focusing on reducing

Table 1.1. Classifications of Variability

Class of Variability	Definition
Clinical Variability	Variability that occurs when different numbers of patients with different conditions present to the healthcare system
Flow Variability	The ebb and flow of patient arrival and discharge within any given time period (day, week, season, etc.)
Professional Variability	The variation in skills and techniques among various healthcare providers

Source: Litvak, E. 2004. "Managing Variability in Patient Flow is the Key to Improving Access to Care, Nursing, Staffing, Quality of Care, and Reducing its Cost." [Online information; retrieved 10/30/06] http://www.iom.edu/Object.File/Master/21/207/

artificial variation provides far more leverage in improving flow than focusing on reducing natural variation.

As we attempt to define flow and how to improve it by measuring and understanding variation, additional classifications of variability can be helpful (Table 1.1).

It is important to recognize that each of these kinds of variability can be reduced using statistical process control tools, which allow us to forecast and predict variation through statistical analysis. The most important tools will be described in this book. An old adage says, "If your only tool is a hammer, every problem is a nail." Similarly, solutions for reducing variability to improve flow will always rely on the use of statistical process control tools and effective leadership techniques such as Toyota's "Lean Management System," which will be described in more detail later. Further, healthcare leaders must be astutely attuned to not only reducing variation, but doing so in a way that delivers the best possible outcome.

> Excellence is what we strive for, but consistency is what we demand.
>
> —Spinoza

While it predated the science of statistical process control and reduction of variation, Spinoza's seventeenth-century philosophical wisdom nonetheless points to the distinction between mere consistency and excellence. For an effective definition of flow, reduction of variation must be augmented by increased predictability and forecasting and a culture of ferocious commitment to innovation. Otherwise, reduced variation alone leaves us without other important flow elements.

A logical extension of flow's reduced variation and increased predictability is the ability to accurately forecast the ability and capacity of the healthcare system and its component subunits. That is, improving flow requires the ability to predict and forecast, within a reasonable degree of certainty, how the system will perform under specific patient volume and acuity loads. For example, many hospitals have adopted a "Green Light, Yellow Light, Red Light" system to identify the bed status for various component units in the hospital, including medical-surgical floors, intensive care units (ICUs), step-down units, and so on. This is an example of using statistical process-control techniques to forecast capacity and flow. Matching capacity to demand is another use of forecasting to impact flow. Using statistical data that are tracked over time, hospitals can predict hours of the day, days of the week, or even seasons of the year when increased patient volume and/or acuity require increased staffing and service capacity.

Predicting variation while simultaneously increasing both predictability and the ability to accurately forecast capacity and capability are thus critically important aspects of the flow definition, yet these elements alone do not completely encompass the features of flow.

3. FLOW AS SYSTEMS THINKING

Popularized by leaders such as Peter Senge (2006), Meg Wheatley (1999), Russ Ackoff (1981), Tom Peters (2003), and others, systems thinking as applied to healthcare relies on an understanding of the fundamental interconnectedness of each of the subprocesses, units, and transfers between elements of the healthcare system. Thus, improving flow within a given healthcare unit (for example, the medical ICU) should be viewed as improving flow within a *subsystem* of the larger healthcare system. While flow may be improved within the medical ICU, it may not translate to an overall improvement in flow for the healthcare system. Indeed, the experience of IHI and others in healthcare flow research indicates that some improvements in flow within subsystems may actually *decrease* flow in other dependent or interconnected areas of the system. For example, if flow improvements in the medical ICU result in faster discharge of patients from the ICU to either step-down or medical-surgical floors, the metrics regarding flow through the ICU are improved. However, if the step-down units have substantial capacity constraints that are not addressed, this may actually worsen flow for these patients) if improving flow is not approached as a systems problem rather than as a sub-system problem. In a similar vein, if early discharge from the ICU to the floor becomes a primary metric, it is important to track the percentage of "bounce-backs," patients who are transferred out of the ICU but are subsequently readmitted to the ICU prior to discharge.

Two subcomponents of systems thinking as it relates to healthcare are *service transitions* and *alignment of incentives*, each of which is addressed in more detail later. As Peter Senge (2006) notes in *The Fifth Discipline: The Art and Practice of the Learning Organization*, two fundamental transitions are necessary to understand systems thinking:

1. a shift from linear cause-effect relationships *to* interrelationships, at many levels, of the subsystems, and
2. seeing processes of change as moving pictures rather than snapshots.

With this view in mind, service transitions and alignment of incentives are clearly essential parts of systems thinking in healthcare, since care of a single patient is provided in various parts of the system, many of which currently operate in functional silos, seemingly without connection or effective communication among them.

A simple example of systems thinking is the increasing reliance on benchmarking or "best in class" approaches, often used in manufacturing but also in service and healthcare industries. Ackoff (1981) points this out in his benchmarking example with regard to automobiles. He notes that the best suspension system may be made by BMW, the best engine by Porsche, the best interior by Rolls Royce, the best frame by General Motors, and the best reliability provided by Toyota. However, if we take the components from each of these manufacturers and try to assemble the "best in class" automobile, not only will the car not run, but it can't even be assembled because the parts don't fit together. (How often does it seem the "parts don't fit together" in your hospital?) Rather, a systems approach is necessary in which the fundamental interrelatedness of processes and services is recognized, measured, and rewarded. This does not diminish the importance of benchmarking as a tool for attaining improved patient flow, but simply accepts its limitations. We should remember the advice of Winston Churchill: "Regardless of how elegant the plans, one must occasionally look at the results."

While viewing healthcare as a fundamentally and functionally interrelated system makes sense, it has not traditionally been viewed as such; therefore, the metrics, risks, and rewards of the system tend to measure and reward subsystems, as opposed to the functionally interrelated system.

Systems Thinking and Service Transitions

Healthcare is one of America's most important and largest industries, one that has a fundamental service aspect. The work of Quint Studer (2004), Len Berry (1999), and Thom Mayer and Robert Cates (2004) has emphasized that healthcare is not just a service business, but a personal service business. Healthcare is delivered person to person, one caregiver or team of caregivers at a time with each patient. Combining and understanding the service nature of healthcare with systems thinking allows us to view healthcare flow as a series of service transitions in which caregivers cooperate in the care of the patient by handing off specific areas of responsibility to other caregivers on the team, much as runners in a relay race seamlessly hand off the baton without losing a stride. Consider the simple example of obtaining a computed tomography (CT) scan of a patient from a medical-surgical floor shown in Figure 1.1.

As the CT process demonstrates, even the most seemingly simple and mundane of healthcare processes embody myriad service hand-offs, from one healthcare provider to another and from one unit or sub-unit to another. Now think about the fact that the physician, nurse, transporter, CT technician, and radiologist (at a minimum) each operate through different reporting structures in the hospital leadership chain. This "functional siloing" effect can have a devastating impact on flow. Unless we manage these service handoffs effectively and proactively, we will never attain consistent and reliable patient flow.

As patients journey through the healthcare system, we should not be surprised if they judge flow by our ability to handle service hand-offs in a way that is thoughtful, integrated, and driven not just toward clinical results, but toward service and system results as well. When thinking of flow as a series of service transitions, remember that first impressions are often lasting impressions. Consider two scenarios of a patient, Mr. Smith, arriving bright and early at patient registration for his elective cardiac catheterization. He says to the registrar, "I'm Bill Smith—I'm here for a cardiac catheterization this morning."

Scenario 1: The registrar, without looking up, shuffles through papers first on her desk, then on the desk behind her, both of which are strewn with paper. She calls to the office staff behind her, "Anyone know about a Smith?" Finally she turns back to the patient and says, "You sure you're in the right place?"

Scenario 2: The registrar rises from her chair, smiles, shakes Mr. Smith's hand, and says, "Mr. Smith, we've been expecting you! Thanks for choosing St. Elsewhere Hospital for your cardiac catheterization. You'll be very satisfied with the care we give."

Figure 1.1 Service Transitions (an example)

Processes

- Physician initiates order for CT scan
  ↓
- CT scheduler documents time and date of availability
  ↓
- Primary nurse makes CT imaging part of daily plan
  ↓
- Transporter arrives on floor, identifies patient in chart, and transports
  ↓
- CT personnel obtains scan, verifies quality of images, and contacts transport
  ↓
- Radiologist interprets scan, enters diagnostic impression, and contacts physician regarding the study
  ↓
- Physician communicates scanned results to the patient

Handoffs

- Unit secretary converts to computer order
  ↓
- Calls/computer message to flow regarding scheduling
  ↓
- Calls/patient transport/radiology for transport
  ↓
- Delivery to CT personnel
  ↓
- Images are displayed for the radiologist
  ↓
- Information is transferred to the chart/physician regarding the study

This example (vastly simplified for our purposes here) shows that the very simple act of obtaining a CT scan can be the source of smooth flow—or disaster when the handoffs are not handled smoothly and efficiently.

On the surface, the same process (initial patient check-in and registration) has occurred. But the experience for the patient is entirely different in Scenario 2 than Scenario 1. Which hospital would you prefer for your healthcare? Which would you prefer to lead?

Here's a simple test to determine whether your institution is attentive to service handoffs as a key component of flow:

> At change of shift, do your nurses walk into the patient's room to introduce the nurse coming on duty, saying, "Mr. Smith, this is Jim, one of my nursing partners. He's going to lead the team delivering your care for the next eight hours—I've briefed him thoroughly about you and he knows your care plan?" Jim then says, "Mr. Smith, I've been looking forward to meeting you. Please let me know if you have any questions at any time."

Is this a consistent experience for your patients? Wouldn't *you* want this to occur if you were the patient?

Alignment of Incentives

Because the healthcare system currently comprises multiple disparate providers converging at the nexus of the acute care hospital, one of the greatest difficulties in improving flow is ensuring that strategic incentives are aligned for these groups of disparate providers. For example, in most acute care settings, members of the medical staff are not employees of the hospital, but are in fact private practitioners whose individual preferences with regard to patient care, the timing of that care, the delivery of that care, and so on, all contribute to artificial professional variation. Unless the strategic incentives for the medical staff can be closely aligned with those of the acute care hospital, improving flow in the acute care setting will be difficult, if not impossible. Further, healthcare leaders must be astutely attuned to not only *reducing variation*, but doing so in a way that delivers the best possible *outcome*.

The situation is further complicated by the fact that, while many healthcare executives understand the importance of aligning incentives at the macroeconomic level (fewer days per case-adjusted admission improves profitability), it is less common to see a deep understanding of the microeconomic or unit-level influence and the fundamental interrelatedness of these areas. For example, the vision, mission, and strategy of the hospital—and its units—should reflect improved flow at the systems level, not just for each of the component units. This is the key element of healthcare leadership for flow: alignment of incentives and commitment to the interrelatedness of healthcare subunits as systems.

Alignment of incentives requires helping everyone in the healthcare system to understand that what they do not only makes a significant difference for their patients, but also has an important impact on the entire system and its profitability. Consider this simple example from the flow frontier, related by a healthcare leader on the front lines, battling to improve flow:

> Our institution had a major commitment toward improving flow and making sure that we were able to view it as the inter-relation of subunits for the good of the patient in a systems approach. An interdisciplinary flow team was formed and a substantial amount of data analysis was done. We looked at "pull" vs. "push" systems, earlier discharge times, hospitalists, and many other factors. And yet we were still not able to have as dramatic an impact on flow as we wanted, particularly as measured by the timeliness of placing patients into beds. We were stuck with minor improvements, and we couldn't even predictably make those.
>
> Finally, at one of the sessions, we were drilling down on the actual process of cleaning the beds, which of course is done by housekeeping. Fortunately, Earl, the director of environmental services, had been invited to the meeting. For nearly an hour, Earl didn't say a word, as he listened to nurses, administrators, and

physicians describe their frustration with not being able to improve flow as dramatically as they had hoped. Finally, there was a lull in the conversation and Earl spoke up: "I can tell you what the problem is. Over 60 percent of the discharges in this hospital occur between 2 p.m. and 3 p.m. At 3 p.m. the current staffing schedule for housekeeping is reduced by half. You've got less than half of the housekeeping force doing the majority of the work, because the people sent home aren't replaced on the 3 p.m. shift."

All of us looked at each other with open mouths and realized the solution was simply to change the staffing pattern of housekeeping!

Matching capacity to demand is one way of aligning strategic incentives, but we must always keep in the mind that it is the entire system whose incentives need to be considered, not just the component parts. Even housekeeping plays a major role in creating flow through alignment of incentives.

4. FLOW AS EMPOWERED PROVIDERS EXCEEDING EXPECTATIONS

Empowered Providers

Empowerment is perhaps one of the most overused and least understood words, not just in healthcare but also in American business and industry. While there are many definitions of empowerment, perhaps the simplest definition is the following:

Empowerment exists to the extent that those charged with the delivery of the service have the freedom to adapt the service to meet the patient/customer needs in real time.

Under this definition, a fundamental question for healthcare providers is, "Tell me about a time you broke the rules on behalf of the patient." This definition helps people understand that, in fact, the frontline service provider, whether the doctor, nurse, lab technician, radiology technician, transporter, or even housekeeper, is the face of the organization to the patient. Thus, each of these providers is a "mini CEO" of the healthcare system and should be appropriately empowered to deliver service within the parameters of the vision and mission statements of the institution, with the freedom to say confidently and caringly to each patient, "*I* will take care of you." This is the principle Jan Carlzon understood when he developed the concept of "moments of truth" (Carlzon 1987). Carlzon stressed that his company, SAS, a Scandinavian airline, had been defining the airline in terms of technical metrics, including revenue capacity, load capacity, profitability, and so on. He stated that he believed the airline was defined by what he described as "50,000 moments of truth a day." A moment of truth occurs when the employees of the company have contact with those they serve—in the airline's case, passengers and the family members accompanying them. In the healthcare system, they are the patients and their families we care for. Carlzon's message, translated to healthcare, is as simple as this: "From the patient's perspective, the people performing this service and delivering the care ARE the company!"

A corollary to empowerment is that exceptional healthcare executives create systems in which each provider at every level is encouraged, indeed rewarded, for making improvements not just in the care and service provided to each patient, but also in the system of care provided. Toyota's Lean Management System is an outstanding example of how providers of products and services are charged with not only excellence in performance, but also excellence in improving the system. At its essence, lean management is the commitment to use less to produce more. The core idea is to accentuate, refine, and improve processes and systems that create value, while eliminating or minimizing non-value-added steps. Truly empowered healthcare employees can use these concepts to topple "functional silos" on behalf of the patient, creating a domino-like reaction that further empowers others as well.

Exceeding Expectations

The sign at Walt Disney World's Space Mountain roller coaster ride reads:

The wait from here is 40 minutes.

Like most Type A, semi-tightly wound healthcare professionals, we immediately set the timer on our watches to see if their estimate is accurate. As masters of the art of "expectation creation and management," the Disney Imagineers artfully subject us to a series of twists and turns as we wind our way through the line, changing scenery often, creating the impression that progress is actually being made. Finally, as we take our seats on the Space Mountain ride and stop the timer—at 34 minutes and 12 seconds—we smugly think, "Terrific, I beat their estimate."

This story illustrates the simple fact that we have expectations in every encounter throughout the course of our day. The genius of the Walt Disney Company is its ability to not only meet but exceed our expectations. Our expectation that we would be on the ride in 40 minutes was bettered by nearly six minutes. (We may actually think we have gotten VIP treatment!) What we don't know is that Disney actively creates the expectation of 40 minutes with the full knowledge that over 98 percent of riders will actually be in their seats on Space Mountain in 32 minutes or less! Their magic in expectation creation certainly works at their parks. In fact, because we exceeded the 32-minute threshold (a threshold that they have set up for themselves, while creating a 40-minute threshold in our minds), Disney's crew was actively deploying additional personnel to help pull the wait down to their target. Thus, Disney *creates* an expectation (40 minutes) that they expect to exceed, then manages that expectation by creating the image that "something is happening; I'm almost there," all the while expecting to exceed the customer's expectation.

In healthcare, flow can be viewed as our ability to anticipate, meet, and exceed the expectations of our patients. We would suggest that healthcare does not currently do this particularly well. For example, how many "The wait from here is 40 minutes" signs do we see in our EDs, radiology suites, or inpatient units? Instead, most of our institutions seem to have an underlying philosophy that "It will take as long as it takes. Now stop bothering me with these questions."

How many institutions script patient encounters? Note how the following scripts improve patient flow, patient safety, and patient satisfaction.

> Mr. Smith, I'm Jenny and I'll be your primary care nurse today. You are on the first day of your hospitalization for heart failure, and we expect to have you home with your family within two days.

> Mr. Jones, I'm Ben and I have been fully briefed on your status during your stay in our hospital. Today you can expect to have a CT scan of your abdomen, an ultrasound examination of your carotid arteries, and a number of lab tests. We will report the results of these tests back to you as soon as we receive them.

> Mrs. Patel, we had hoped to be able to pull your chest tube today, but there is still an air leak, which means that we need to leave it in for another 24 hours. At that point, we will reevaluate and keep you informed every step of the way. I'm sorry that this happened, but we hope this won't prolong your hospital stay any longer than necessary. I'd be happy to explain this to your husband either by phone or when he comes in to visit.

These conversations occur far less frequently than they should in our healthcare systems, simply because we have not done as good a job as we should at educating staff on the needs of anticipating, meeting, and exceeding patient expectations as a way of attaining excellence in patient flow.

How can we discover patients' flow expectations? In two words: Ask them!

While healthcare systems need to research patient expectations more carefully, this can in fact be done at the bedside every single day that we care for patients. We can simply say, "Mr. Smith, I'm Jim, your primary care nurse today. What are your expectations for your hospital stay?" The same question can be asked for primary care visits, outpatient surgeries, ED visits, or whatever aspect of healthcare is being delivered. It is certainly difficult if not impossible to meet expectations, much less exceed them, if we don't have a clear statement of what those expectations are.

What is the difference between *meeting* and *exceeding* expectations? The issue of patients' and families' questions regarding care provides a simple and concise example. Consider these two scenarios, both of which use scripts in dealing with expectations:

Emergency department RN to patient: "Do you have any other questions? Just ask me. I have plenty of time.

E-mail from primary care physician to patient: "I noticed you have an office appointment next week. I want to be sure to answer any questions you may have, so please e-mail them to me so that I can review them prior to your visit.

The first script is an example of meeting expectations, since we know patients in fact will have questions; this script uses, as Quint Studer (2004) refers to it, "the right words at the right time from the right person to the right patient." The e-mail example is an example of *exceeding* expectations, since very few physicians utilize e-mail effectively to determine the needs and expectations of their patients *in advance*. The same sort of communication, whether by e-mail, voice mail, or telephone, can be used for scheduled healthcare visits to any part of the system, including outpatient surgery, inpatient elective surgery, cardiac catheterization, and so on. Further, the e-mail survey is a vastly underused tool for rediscovering patient expectations and determining whether they were met during the course of the healthcare visit.

5. FLOW AS DEMAND CAPACITY MANAGEMENT

Matching service supply (or capacity) to service (or patient) demand presents a fascinating and crucial challenge. Service capacity is a perishable commodity—it cannot be stored. For example, an airplane flying with empty seats has lost forever the opportunity of filling those particular seats on that particular flight and collecting revenue for those potential additional passengers. A surgical suite with a full crew that goes unused has lost that service opportunity forever. An ED that remains idle and unused for two hours cannot use that capacity when or if there is a sudden influx of patients, as much as they would like to.

Much of what we think of as service or clinical capacity is determined or fixed by decisions made in advance of the day of service delivery (and often long in advance of the day of service). These decisions are usually made on the basis of historical demand. Using these data, and availing ourselves of the tool of forecasting, we attempt to match capacity to demand. (More on forecasting—a critical tool and skillset that is woefully underused in healthcare—in Chapter 5.) We often base our decisions on average demand instead of peak demand, and we often fail to take the variation in demand into account.

A service is both produced and consumed (or used) at the same time. Unlike products stored in warehouses for future consumption, a service is an intangible personal experience that cannot be transferred from one person to another or saved for a rainy day. Contrast this with Home Depot and the demand for lawn mowers, for example. If Home Depot expects to sell 20 lawn mowers this week, but fails to do so, the store can simply hold the mowers to meet next week's demand. Service opportunity, however, once lost is lost forever.

Matching demand and service capacity is a critical component of flow and requires a number of tools, strategies, and interventions. It is critical to our success, much has been learned, and there remain countless opportunities for innovation. We will explore data-driven decisions: adjusting staff, space, and service to demand; planning for contingencies; and implementing creative solutions to difficult patient flow problems later in the book.

THE FLOW MASTER MATRIX™:
CONNECTING AND CREATING FLOW

The final lens through which flow can be viewed is the connectivity of these five lenses. Each of the five components of flow is an important element of the definition, yet no one element, in and of itself, is complete. As philosophers and theologians might say:

> Each is a necessary condition for flow (it must be present for flow to occur) but none is a sufficient condition for flow (no one element is enough to guarantee flow).

In other words, only the connectivity of the component elements of the definition truly enable flow to occur. To be sure, not every element need be present for an idea or initiative to improve flow. And yet the more elements of the definition there are present, the more likely the initiative will improve flow.

The final component of the flow definition is creativity. In his book, *Flow: The Psychology of Optimal Experience*, the great sociologist Mihaly Csikszentmihalyi (1990) helped define the flow phenomenon that positively affects people's lives. He noted, "Flow cannot be pursued—it must ensue."

In healthcare, we must understand the definition of flow; educate our leadership and management teams in the component parts thereof; form the vision for flow in our institutions; place our imprimatur on the effort; and ensure that the will, ideas, and tools for execution are present so that flow can ensue. As we will demonstrate in detail, a clear set of flow metrics and measurements must exist to determine the extent to which flow has been attained. *Yet the healthcare executive's role in improving flow is primarily one of creating the conditions under which flow can occur.*

Finally, what is the relationship of flow to other critically important elements of healthcare leadership, including patient safety, customer satisfaction, employee satisfaction, risk reduction, high reliability, and so on? Simply stated, flow is related to each of these aspects in that organizations that have been able to optimize flow have seen dramatic improvements in each of these areas, as well as in profitability. Thus, improving flow improves each of these areas that are so critical for success in today's healthcare environment. If patient safety, customer satisfaction, employee satisfaction, risk reduction, and profitability are our destination in healthcare, then improving flow is the vehicle that takes us on the journey.

References

Ackoff, R. 1981. *Creating the Corporate Future*. St. Louis, MO: John Wiley and Sons.

Berry, L. L. 1999. *Discovering the Soul of Service: The Nine Drivers of Sustainable Business Success*. New York: The Free Press.

Carlzon, J. 1987. *Moments of Truth: New Strategies for Today's Customer-Driven Economy*. New York: HarperCollins.

Csikszentmihalyi, M. 1990. *Flow: The Psychology of Optimal Experience—Steps Toward Enhancing the Quality of Life*. New York: Harper and Row.

Haraden, C., and R. Resar. 2004. "Patient Flow in Hospitals: Understanding and Controlling It Better." *Frontiers of Health Services Management* 20 (4): 3–15.

Institute for Healthcare Improvement. 2003. *Optimizing Patient Flow: Moving Patients Smoothly Through Acute Care Settings*. Boston: IHI.

Litvak, E., P. I. Buerhaus, and F. Davidoff. 2005. "Managing Unnecessary Variability." *Journal on Quality and Patient Safety* 31 (6): 330–339.

Mayer, T. A., and R. J. Cates. 2004. *Leadership for Great Customer Service: Satisfied Patients, Satisfied Employees*. Chicago: Health Administration Press.

Peters, T. 2003. *Re-Imagine!* London: Dorling Kindersley.

Senge, P. M. 2006. *The Fifth Discipline: The Art and Practice of the Learning Organization*. New York: Doubleday.

Studer, Q. 2004. *Service Excellence*. Baltimore, MD: Firestarter Press.

Wheatley, M. 1999. *Leadership and the New Science: Discovering Order in a Chaotic World*. San Francisco: Berrit-Koehler.

CHAPTER 2

The Benefits of Flow

THE COMPLEX PROCESS through which a hospital admits, treats, and discharges patients requires the delicate orchestration of staff and services. The success of this orchestration—flow—can be gauged in patient safety and satisfaction, staff satisfaction and stability, administrative smoothness, and the organization's bottom line. The key to an optimally functioning hospital lies in all these factors working together. If patients wait seven hours in the ED for an inpatient bed or three hours in the discharge queue or spend an extra day or two in the hospital waiting for test results to be interpreted and acted on, their care is compromised and they are unhappy. Patients who have a choice, often the discriminating and insured patients, may vote with their feet and leave for another hospital or treatment option. If patients are pleased with their experience, however, they return and tell their friends and neighbors. If staff are happy with the working conditions, they remain loyal and recommend the hospital to other potential employees. A smoothly running hospital with an effective, committed workforce that serves a satisfied community of patients is an administrator's nirvana, and the bottom line reflects the system's success.

With all the potential for wins, managing and improving patient flow is an opportunity no healthcare organization can afford to miss. From one perspective, improving patient flow focuses on reducing waiting times for patients to be served—treated in the ED, admitted to the hospital, taken to radiology or the lab, or discharged from the hospital. Yet the ramifications of this seemingly simple aspect of flow are far-reaching. The same long wait that frustrates, frightens, infuriates, or even endangers patients creates tremendous stress for the people in the system who are delivering these services, including the nurses, physicians, and hospital leaders who are accountable for the quality of care the hospital delivers. What does this mean? It means that the cost of a bottleneck in the system is paid in the areas of patient safety and satisfaction; staff stability, attitude, and quality of service; and, ultimately, the hospital's bottom line, since poor flow reduces the system's functional capacity to provide care. That's the bad news.

The good news is that we own the system we use and we have the power to change it. When he observes that "every system is perfectly designed to achieve the results it achieves," Don Berwick (1996) of IHI suggests both the inertia of any existing system and its inherent potential for retrofit. If patients are stacked in the halls in our EDs, if it takes days to get advanced diagnostic studies read and hours to get our x-rays back from radiology, if surgical schedules are overbooked, if ambulances are diverted to other hospitals from our doors, our system of patient flow is *designed* for these outcomes. This means two things:

1. We ourselves enable and sustain an ineffective system for moving patients through our hospitals.
2. To get a different result, we need to change the system.

Will change be easy? No. Will it be worth the effort? Yes. To begin, we need three tools for improving flow—will, ideas, and execution (Figure 2.1). With these tools in hand, it is up to us to improve the flow. When we do, everybody wins.

Figure 2.1. The Three Tools of Flow Improvement

Will	• Clear, Unrelenting Commitment • Repeated Expression of That Commitment • Support of Initiatives
Ideas	• Toolkit Contents such as Fast Track, Flow Team, Adopt-a-Boarder, etc.
Execution	• Metrics-Based Management • Unwavering Support

HOW PATIENTS WIN

Patients are the frontline beneficiaries of efficient patient flow. They receive better care and better service in a healthcare system in which commitment to good flow reduces chaos and delays. Patients are coming to the hospital better informed than ever before and have higher expectations about both safety and service. They no longer passively trust the provider to have all the answers and often want to participate more actively in decisions about their care. At the same time, patients also demand more accountability on the part of the provider and will often expect compensation if something goes wrong.

> The baby boomers are the largest consumers of healthcare today—and the baby boomers always get their way!
> —Tom Peters (2005)

The baby boom generation demands more information and attention than that which their parents accepted as the norm. For example, an older friend laughs about being left waiting in the maternity ward all night because the nurses changed shifts right after his daughter was born and nobody thought to tell him the news.

Now there's a flow problem! Yet what was accepted without complaint in 1956 is hardly likely to be tolerated now. With healthcare a high-dollar item in most patients' budgets, a sense of entitlement has eroded the earlier deferential patient–provider dynamic. Patients have more healthcare choices, and perception of safety and service helps drive those choices. In short, for the benefit of patient safety, clinical outcomes, and patient satisfaction, the time has come to pay closer attention to patient flow throughout the healthcare system.

Patient Safety

Good flow enhances patient safety by both reducing the risk of medical errors and enabling timely delivery of care. Smooth flow creates a climate of predictability, communication, and reliability in which the healthcare team can do what they do best—take care of patients.

Reduced Medical Error

Patient safety is every hospital's highest priority, and it has been estimated that 1 in 1,000 admitted patients suffers significantly from an adverse event in the hospital. Healthcare clinical processes currently operate in an environment where in 1 to 10 percent of occurrences, there is a failure in care (i.e., the process does not occur exactly the way it is intended). High occupancy and overcrowding are associated with higher adverse event rates and higher morbidity and mortality. In 1999 the Institute of Medicine issued a report that alleged that medical error was responsible for almost 100,000 deaths each year of hospitalized patients in the United States (Corrigan and Kohn 2000). This report, *To Err Is Human: Building a Safer Health System*, jump-started a very public effort in medical centers and hospitals across the country to improve patient safety. Several articles have challenged this allegation on statistical principles, but nevertheless, medical error has to be acknowledged and it is receiving considerable media attention.

The publicity surrounding the issue of medical error fuels a growing public fear that healthcare institutions are somehow unsafe. Patients have concerns about such issues as drug-resistant bacteria, medication errors, and wrong-site surgery. With half of all hospitalized patients now entering the healthcare system through the perceived chaos of the ED, and with 80 percent of hospital EDs at overcapacity at some time during the day, that patients are anxious about their own safety is not surprising. Hospital errors or lapses in care often result from the staff's exhaustion from dealing with stacked-up patients. Paul Duke, an ED nurse who wrote an opinion piece in the February 2, 2004, issue of *Newsweek*, summarized the problem: "I'm so overworked that I go home at night praying I haven't made a mistake that might hurt someone."

While Duke is commenting in the context of the acute shortage of nurses, his statement points toward the cost of overextending staff: extreme and constant stress, which makes errors more likely. Reducing the variation that wastes time and creates communication gaps makes the hospital safer. When staff are not working at a breakneck pace to keep up with an overload of patients, they can devote more time to caring for each patient and to maintaining clear communication with each other.

When patient flow is expeditious, seamless, planned, and monitored, patients and their families perceive the hospital as a safe and a caring place to be. Patient flow initiatives that help accomplish this goal are being well received by patients and by staff. For example, in the Full Capacity Protocol developed at Stony Brook Medical Center in New York, admitted patients are moved from the hallways of the ED to the hallways of the units upstairs when the ED is full. Similarly, the Adopt-a-Boarder protocol developed first at Inova Fairfax Hospital in Falls Church, Virginia, creates a threshold-based system for medical-surgical floors to accept hospital boarders when capacity has been overloaded.

These protocols, versions of which are being increasingly adopted around the country, help reduce demands on ED staff and services and provide patients with better-quality care in a quieter setting than ED hallways. The Stony Brook staff, currently presenting their concept around the country, have photographs of patient boarding in the ED and in the hospital hallways. These pictures compellingly illustrate the difference between the crowded and frenetic ED and the quiet, controlled setting of the ward.

Preserved Access to Care

Controlling flow to reduce overcrowding in the ED also helps keep the hospital open to receive patients. Ambulance diversion, especially from trauma centers, decreases chances for recovery or survival in patients diverted to other hospitals. Contrary to popular belief, diversion is not a regional but rather a national phenomenon. A 2001 government study reported that more than 75 million Americans living in 22 states are affected by ambulance diversions, which impede access to care (McCraig 2006). A study completed by the University of Texas at Houston School of Public Health in November 2002 found that the mortality rate of trauma patients doubled when both Level 1 trauma centers in Houston were on diversion for eight or more hours (Save Our Emergency Rooms 2002). Avoiding diversion, therefore, is much more than a resource-management strategy—it can mean life or death for critically ill patients.

Improved Clinical Outcomes

Good flow enhances patient safety by enabling timely response to clinical conditions. Patients have a better chance of good clinical outcomes when some procedures are done within a certain time-frame. Even less sophisticated healthcare consumers are increasingly aware that good healthcare is "on the clock." With the growing transparency of data in healthcare and the advent of web sites like Hospitalcompare.com, consumers can now track the performance of hospitals in attending to these time-dependent conditions. The data are compelling and widely accepted for several important conditions:

- For acute myocardial infarction (AMI), outcomes are better if the patient either receives thrombolytic therapy within 30 minutes or gets to the cardiac catheterization lab within 90 minutes.
- Patients who have community-acquired pneumonia have better outcomes when antibiotics are administered within four hours of arrival.
- Patients suffering from acute stroke have better outcomes when they receive timely care, often including thrombolytic therapy, by a stroke team.

The concept of Rapid Response Teams, promoted by the Institute for Healthcare Improvement (IHI 2005), is also gaining popularity and typifies the ongoing efforts being made to improve on the "timeliness of care" goal by anticipating and interrupting downward clinical spirals, which are indicated by changes in clinical appearances and clinical markers.

Patient Satisfaction

While certainly not a life-or-death issue, good flow improves patient satisfaction with the overall healthcare experience. As we have noted already, patients are not only patients but customers as well. Therefore, we want to anticipate patient expectations and design flow into care processes to meet or exceed those expectations.

Caring Service
As the first chapter makes clear, flow is much more than turnaround times or the rate at which patients are moved through the system. Flow is the way the patients are moved as well, with emphasis on caring service. In a hospital with good flow, the healthcare team places a high priority on communication with patients and families, and waiting times are reduced and explained. Providers are empowered to adapt

the service to meet the patients' needs in real time. Because the frontline service provider—the doctor, the nurse, the lab technician, the housekeeper—is the face of the organization to the patient, he or she can say confidently and caringly to the patient, "I will take care of you." In a hospital with good flow, such empowerment is key to breaking through service silos and meeting patients' needs.

Reduced and Informed Waits

During the past 15 years, an explosion of patient satisfaction research has helped to define good customer service in healthcare. At the forefront is the realization that wait times and the perception of wait times correlate with patient satisfaction; thus, patients respond favorably to anything that shortens stays and up-front waits. Being made to wait makes a patient feel neglected, especially if he or she remains unacknowledged or uninformed during that time. While long waits are certainly not the only cause of patient complaints, delays in service do influence patients' perceptions of the quality of their care and indicate an overstressed system and staff. In this environment, service lapses are more likely.

Both service intervals and the perception of those intervals are important. This is where the Walt Disney Company's concept of "expectation creation," discussed in the first chapter, comes in. When the ED patient flow system moves patients quickly to a care area where they are evaluated by a physician in a timely fashion (less than 30 minutes is the accepted service quality goal), patients perceive that wait times are acceptable. When the time interval from triage to physician evaluation increases, the rate of patients who leave without being seen (a dramatic indicator of patient dissatisfaction) goes up linearly. Innovations such as bedside registration (which can be implemented with a registration clerk and a clipboard, where bedside computers are lacking) and treatment teams improve satisfaction because they effectively get the physician to the bedside sooner—the most critical time interval from the patient's point of view. Also, tracking door-to-doctor times and overall lengths of stay as well as sharing data with practitioners through a comprehensive continuous quality improvement program can reduce time intervals. Further, using metric-based management—for example, implementing bedside registration and tracking door-to-doctor intervals—has been shown to reduce throughput times and improve patient satisfaction.

Smoothing surgical flow, discussed in Chapter 3 and elsewhere, has tremendous capacity to improve patient flow and increase bed turns. The waits and delays on the hospital floor or in specialized units for diagnostic test results, special procedures, and handoffs of information offer rich opportunities for improved flow and reduced waits.

Managed Waits

Waiting is a part of life in the modern world, and increasingly researchers are bringing their insights to this realm of subjective experience. Armed with data and a new understanding about the psychology of waiting, some organizations are "managing the waits" involved at their facilities quite deftly (for example, Disney and Ritz-Carlton). Healthcare systems with good flow adapt strategies from service-oriented businesses to improve their patients' wait experience.

Before looking at the psychology of waiting as it pertains to the healthcare setting, there are two laws of service worth noting. First, if the service provided exceeds the customer's expectations, the customer will be satisfied. The converse is also true: if service does not meet expectations, then the customer will likely be dissatisfied. Second, it is hard to play catch-up, so if the service encounter begins with unmet expectations, improving on the patient's perceptions later on is difficult. The restaurant industry routinely employs these principles, deliberately promising a wait time in excess of the true "expected time." Thus, customers are pleased to be seated earlier than expected and have a more positive feeling as they begin their meals.

For the benefit of waiting patients and their families, good flow systems address and exploit principles of the psychology of waiting (Maister 1985). These principles are listed in Figure 2.2.

Figure 2.2. The Psychology of Waiting

1. Occupied time feels shorter than unoccupied time.

2. People want to get started.

3. Anxiety makes waits seem longer.

4. Uncertain waits are longer than known, finite waits.

5. Unexplained waits are longer than explained waits.

6. Unfair waits are longer than equitable waits.

7. The more valuable the service, the longer the customer will wait.

8. Solo waits feel longer than group waits.

Armed with an understanding of how patients experience the wait for hospital services, systems committed to good flow make these wait times more tolerable by the use of informed waits, filling the time with instructive or distracting material, such as television and instructional videos. Patients and their families are kept occupied and informed through various means, some of which are listed in Figure 2.3.

These methods that make inevitable waiting less anxiety-inducing and burdensome increase patient satisfaction. Bursch, Beezy, and Shaw (1993) have shown that perceived waiting time, as opposed to actual waiting time, is the most important variable contributing to patient satisfaction, a finding that has been replicated by others. The data correlating patient waits with patient satisfaction are irrefutable.

A Patient Satisfaction Success Story

LDS Hospital is a 520-bed tertiary care and trauma center affiliated with the University of Utah School of Medicine. It serves as a referral trauma center for a three-state region, as a cardiovascular center with open-heart capabilities, and as a neurosurgical and transplant center. Its ED has the highest case-mix index and acuity in Utah. No residency in emergency medicine is currently offered; however, medical students and residents are present in the

Figure 2.3. Tools for Managing Wait Times

Concept of Psychology of Waiting	Intervention
Occupy time	• TVs, magazines, health information • Company (friends, family) • Healthcare forms
Start process	• Direct to room • Advanced triage/Advanced intervention • Team triage
Manage Anxiety	• Treat both the customer service diagnosis and clinical diagnosis • Use scripts
Certainty	• Previews—anticipated delays • Green–yellow–red system • Let delays and causes be known
Explanation	• In-process previews and scripts • Keep family members informed
Equitable delays	• Announce reasons for delays • Address "fairness" issues • Address level of acuity
Value of service	• The value equation • Maximize benefits • Minimize burdens
Group waits	• Visitors • Family

hospital on all general and specialty services. These residents also complete clinical rotations in the ED. This is not typically an environment conducive to the quality improvement/customer service ideology and metrics, for such teaching hospitals often perform worse in those areas than a community hospital of the same size.

In 1998, the annual ED patient census at LDS Hospital was near 28,000, of which 20 percent were admitted. The intensive care unit admission rate was also very high, usually over 20 percent of total ED admissions, reflecting the acuity of the patient population. The ED had two major resuscitation areas: a two-bed medical resuscitation area and a two-bed trauma resuscitation area, with adjacent dedicated conventional radiography and computed tomography suites. There were 23 room beds, 15 of which were monitored; additionally, 7 hallway stretchers had become permanent patient care areas. The ED was "paperless," with historical records, nurse charting, respiratory therapy charting, radiography, laboratory, and outpatient clinic charting all available in electronic format. There were computer terminals at every bed, and another eight terminals at the central workstation. All radiographs of any modality were digitized, and the ED had two viewing stations. The hospital and its parent organization, Intermountain Health Care (IHC), had a widely known history of quality improvement projects and decision-support technologies.

Despite this background and numerous technological innovations, the department faced mounting problems. The original physical space was designed to accommodate 18,000 visits per year of much lower acuity, but rapid increases in volume led to poor turnaround times and departmental process inefficiencies. The department had high patient complaint ratios, high walk-away rates, and poor patient satisfaction scores.

A comprehensive quality improvement program was instituted that included feedback to physicians and staff regarding throughput, the fastidious monitoring of metrics, and the institution of a bedside registration system. As can be seen in Figure 2.4, the

Figure 2.4. LDS Hospital: Mean Turnaround Time by Quarter

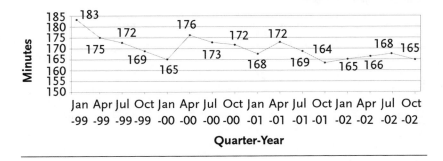

Figure 2.5. LDS Hospital: Emergency Department Complaints by Year

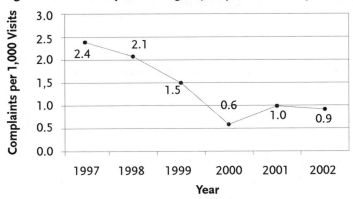

throughput times improved steadily over the four-year period after the program's inception. Concomitantly, the rate of complaints and the number of walk-aways (in this sample, the patients leaving against medical advice and patients leaving without being seen) fell steadily (Figures 2.5 and 2.6).

During the same period the hospital administration commissioned patient satisfaction surveys for the ED by an outside agency. The results show a steady improvement in patient satisfaction (Figure 2.7).

By attending to patient flow issues and improving the throughput of ED patients, this department, an unlikely laboratory for

The Benefits of Flow   33

Figure 2.6. LDS Hospital: Rate of Patients Leaving Against Medical Advice or Without Being Seen

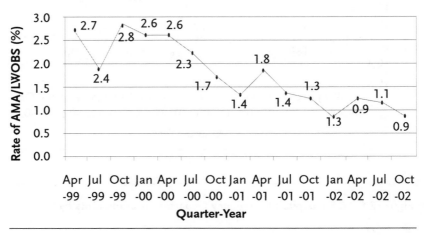

Figure 2.7. LDS Hospital: Patient Satisfaction Survey Results

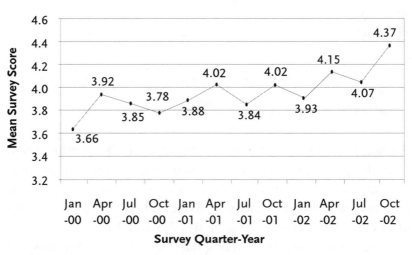

Patient Satisfaction Service Quality Scale: 3 = Good; 4 = Very Good; 5 = Excellent

patient satisfaction efforts, demonstrated gains in terms of patient satisfaction. The ultimate expression of ED patient dissatisfaction (walk-away rates) showed the most dramatic improvement. *The most compelling reason to embark on patient flow work is for the sake of patients and their perceptions of their healthcare experience.*

HOW THE HEALTHCARE TEAM WINS

As Peter Drucker (1994) observes, hospitals are the most complex of the modern knowledge organizations. The tempo of work today is not only faster but also more unpredictable, which presents enormous challenges. In a hospital that focuses on the contribution of clinical activities to the mission of patient care, there is little difficulty in achieving teamwork. Members of the team may change and leadership can shift between individuals, yet the quality of that teamwork never varies. Where this commitment and discipline are lacking, one sees a group of individual caregivers rather than a high-performance team. Patient flow suffers, clinical quality suffers, and there is greater employee dissatisfaction and turnover.

Each member of the care team must come to the job or role with a perspective or conception of how the job works, gleaned from the culture of the hospital. Culture is a shared, learned, or symbolic system of values, beliefs, and attitudes that shapes and influences perception and behavior. In other words, it is "the way we do things around here." If poor patient flow has become an accepted norm, or if communication or conflict between administration and staff, between team members, or between hospital subsystems is part of the culture ("fighting in the cockpit"), team members are ultimately unable to deliver optimal care. Exhausted, angry, disappointed, anxious, distracted, or detached staff members cannot fulfill their roles with the commitment to service that is optimal for excellence in patient care.

Team members ask themselves each day, "How will things go today?" "How will I perform?" "What is my role in patient care?"

"What will I accomplish?" In a hospital with a chronic logjam of patients, the morale of administrators, physicians, nurses, and support staff can wear down in a hurry. The demands of constant crisis, with attendant breakdowns in communication, us-versus-them mentalities, and feelings of never being able to gain control create a climate in which people cannot do their best work. People go into healthcare because they want to make a difference. They want to create value and meaning in their lives and in the workplace. When they are forced to practice in an environment that does not allow them to deliver high-quality care, they become enormously frustrated, which affects morale and fosters learned helplessness, lethargy, and fatigue. This is not an environment conducive to the kind of care that you want your patients or your family to receive, nor is it the kind of reputation for care that you want in your community.

On the other hand, a healthcare setting with smooth patient flow fosters workforce satisfaction. For the healthcare team as well as for the patients, effective patient flow improves the quality of life. Before implementing any change, we should ask two questions: "Is it good for the patients?" and "Is it good for the healthcare team?" Patient flow has a tremendous impact on job satisfaction and quality of service for all members of the healthcare team. A good patient flow plan benefits staff in numerous ways.

Empowerment

Good patient flow plans benefit staff by creating an environment in which it is easy to do the right thing. Competent and committed staff are empowered to meet patient needs. Positive empowerment builds confidence and is seen by staff as a measure of perceived value to the employer. Empowerment also makes the job easier by breaking down the silos that make it harder to get the right things done. Empowerment is an essential aspect of hospital flow.

Effective Team Formation

Good flow systems enable, even demand, effective teamwork. Members who lack commitment to the excellent-service agenda must be remotivated, retrained, or reassigned. Work is a more enjoyable experience if we are surrounded by others who share our goals and are pleasant and easy to work with. Trust, accountability, civility, and respect characterize effective team interactions. It is no fun apologizing to patients for a team member's rude treatment or putting up with selfish or disrespectful attitudes as we try to work together. Good commitment to flow precludes tolerance of these and other behaviors that impede quality improvement efforts.

A Teamwork Story

A hospital consultant in a big hurry was zipping down a North Carolina back road on a rainy afternoon. When he hit a puddle that was just a little too deep, his Mercedes skidded off the road, landing neatly in a shallow ditch. Fortunately, there was a farmhouse nearby, so he walked over, knocked on the door, and asked the farmer for help. "Sure, I'll help you," the old farmer said. "Just let me go get my plough horse, Buddy."

When they had gotten to the car and hooked everything up, the farmer leaned over and said to the horse, "Pull, Bessie, pull!" Nothing happened. The farmer leaned over again and said, "Pull, Mabel, pull!" Again nothing happened. The farmer leaned over again and said, "Pull, Flossie, pull!" And again nothing happened. Then the farmer leaned over and whispered, "Pull, Buddy, pull!" Buddy's shoulders strained against the harness as he hauled the Mercedes out of the ditch. The consultant turned to the farmer and said, "You just called your horse by the wrong name three times." "Naw, I didn't," he replied. "Old Buddy is blind, and if he thought he was doing this all by himself there'd be no way he would ever start pulling!"

What's the point? It's wonderful to have a team. As we have mentioned before, there is a clear distinction between a group of individuals and a team. Team members should feel that others are "pulling their weight" and that "we are all in this together." Sometimes we just have to get ourselves pulling in the necessary direction first. A clear understanding of team formation, team dynamics, and leading teams through change is essential to creating and sustaining flow. The works of John Kotter (1996), Tom Peters (2005), and Badaracco and Ellsworth (1989) provide a good starting point.

Better Support for Nurses and Caregivers

Keys to establishing a positive staff experience include creating time with the patient and a positive environment in which to work. Improving flow can create that time. In the early years, for example, nurses were trained by religious organizations to be nurturers. Caring for people was the hallmark of the profession. The satisfaction that resulted from this experience helped to draw good nurses to the profession and kept them there. In the current environment, however, nurses have often become technical and task specialists who may have little time for connecting with and nurturing patients. This situation creates an environment high in frustration and low in career satisfaction.

In an effort to address the interrelated issues of the nursing shortage, the scarcity of experienced nurses, and the frustrations and lack of job satisfaction among emergency nurses, BestPractices, Inc., surveyed these nurses at a Level 1 trauma center (BestPractices, Inc. 2005). The survey was intended to identify which nursing roles and duties were most and least satisfying on an ordinal scale. Perhaps not surprisingly, chart documentation and technical procedures (blood draws, IV starts, suctioning, etc.) were least satisfying, while patient interaction, counseling, and diagnostic evaluation were among the most satisfying. Using these data, the group created a pilot program that focused on using senior ED nurses to supervise teams of more junior nurses, who in turn supervise groups of ED "Super Techs." The ED "Super Techs" are emergency medical technicians and paramedics who perform some procedures previously performed by nurses. Documentation duties have been simplified by using either scribes (college students who document for the nurses and/or physicians) or electronic medical records. While the results of this project are preliminary, the initial data indicate that both patient flow and satisfaction have improved, and employee satisfaction has risen dramatically as well.

Flow-centered teamwork that extends beyond the silos of the ICU, the ED, or the operating room fosters mutual support among members of the care team and across the system. Reducing wasted time and communication failures that create frustration and fuel conflicts provides opportunity for better caregiving. Staff are united and empowered to make decisions that are best for the patient. Positively improving flow in your hospital attracts and keeps good staff, which in turn translates into more time available for each patient. For example, in 1997 the ED at Nash General Hospital in North Carolina had a 33 percent RN vacancy rate and an overwhelmed, overworked staff. A year later, after patient flow initiatives had been implemented, 11 nurses within the hospital system were waiting to come to work in the ED. Changing the environment by improving flow processes and by training and grooming the staff resulted in positive attitudes and transformed the ED for both workers and patients.

Good flow systems—such as a minimally demanding call structure, manageable shift durations, and a healing environment that is clean, spacious, and feels good to staff as well as patients—establish conditions that support caregivers. Effective communication is both a necessary component and a consequence of flow. In a good flow system, hospital leaders understand the perspective of each team member, and team members understand the perspective of the patient and the healthcare institution. The care team is organized and bound around a common purpose.

Rewards and Incentives

Effective flow initiatives provide staff with incentives and rewards for contributions to positive patient flow in the hospital. These rewards range from the tangible—movie tickets for a service compliment from a difficult patient, a bonus for a time-saving idea—to the intangible—personal acknowledgment by the leaders and supervisors, and department recognition. Healthcare workers in good flow systems enjoy committed leadership from the top, with administrators who walk the walk—that is, show up at the point of service, frequently offer words of support and acknowledgment, and give financial and administrative support to flow incentives.

Team structures can be designed to reward staff as well. Leadership provides strategic direction, monitors the performance of the team, teaches, and enables hands-on treatment of the patient. For example, individual team members may cycle on and off the team and work shifts of differing lengths. The flow structure makes it possible to pass the baton—a smooth orchestration of people focused on the clearly defined goal of providing quality and caring service in a positive work environment.

An undeniable connection exists between patient satisfaction and staff satisfaction. This continuum makes sense because a better working environment for the staff translates into more (and more pleasant) attention to the patients. Results of Press-Ganey surveys in which patient and staff satisfaction were measured show a clear relationship between the two, and at one hospital, while customer satisfaction increased, employee turnover decreased by 57 percent (Press 2002). When team members work in a climate of clearly articulated, shared goals, with the tools to accomplish those goals, the workplace becomes a more satisfying place to be. With today's significant shortage of skilled healthcare workers, especially nurses, the relationships between flow and workforce retention, longevity, and satisfaction (and, in turn, patient satisfaction) are well worth noting and mining.

HOW ADMINISTRATORS WIN

Opportunity's favorite disguise is trouble.

—Frank Tyger

From an administrative perspective, managing and improving patient flow through the ED and through inpatient settings makes an enormous amount of sense. In terms of patient safety and satisfaction, workforce stability, regulatory requirements, and the healthcare system bottom line, a culture focused on optimizing patient flow will realize gains on a variety of fronts. While we have already covered the wins from the patient and healthcare team perspectives, more is still to be gained.

Risk Reduction

From a patient safety standpoint, well-managed patient flow means less chaos and attendant risk of error in the delivery of medical services. While the benefits for patients in a reduced-risk environment speak for themselves, benefits for administrators accrue as well. Medical error carries high costs in lawsuit settlements and damage to a healthcare system's reputation that translates into lost referrals to the hospital and patients choosing other health systems for services. Reducing risk to patients is a compelling benefit of good flow initiatives.

The ED is now widely recognized as one critical area (the others being surgery and surgical admissions) in which to begin addressing the challenges of hospital flow. While the ED is not the source of flow problems, healthcare system backup typically results in ED overcrowding and the boarding of patients, which in turn make the delivery of safe care a serious challenge. From the timely administration of antibiotics to rapid cardiac catheterization during an acute cardiac ischemic event, evidence-based clinical guidelines are growing in emergency medicine. Efficient and accurate implementation of these guidelines, along with optimal clinical outcomes, requires smooth patient flow. Furthermore, a growing body of data indicates that simply moving boarders out of the ED can shorten their hospital length of stay (probably because intensive appropriate care begins on a unit equipped for those clinical problems)(Sprivulis et al. 2006; Cameron 2006; Richardson 2006). The ED can't do everything as well as the inpatient units can, and it shouldn't be expected to. Smoothing patient flow in the operating room with the attendant admissions to the postanesthesia care unit (PACU) and intensive care unit (ICU) also leads to concomitant improvements in patient safety, service, and workforce satisfaction.

Patient Satisfaction

Waits and delays are a frequent source of patient dissatisfaction and complaints, often costing healthcare systems time and money to resolve. It has been estimated that a single complaint may cost an institution on the order of $8,000 in terms of lost business, waived billings, and lost wages (i.e., paying workers who could be performing other tasks to investigate the complaint and to minimize any ill effects) (See chapter 3. figures 3.3 and 3.4).

When waits and delays create flow problems, the ED may lose patients by two mechanisms. First, as delays to see a physician mount, patients who have other healthcare options (typically patients with insurance) may leave as walk-aways. Walk-aways are patients who

- leave without being seen (LWBS);
- leave without treatment (LWOT);
- leave before treatment is complete (LBTC); or
- leave against medical advice (AMA).

These patients are often complaints personified. Even though they may not verbally complain, their actions indicate dissatisfaction with wait times. Such patients are also known to put the institution at risk in terms of liability and are usually tracked closely by quality or risk-management departments at the institutional level. Second, the ED loses potential patients because of the department's reputation for long waits. People who are dissatisfied with wait times spread the word among family, friends, and coworkers.

Revenue and Financial Viability

While overcrowding creates administrative headaches from satisfaction and safety perspectives, overcrowding has other costs as well. When overcrowding forces an ED to go on diversion, the costs are easily calculable. Ambulance arrivals are more likely to need admission than the walk-in population, and a hospital admission generates a financial return in the neighborhood of $6,000 to $8,000. Therefore, from a strictly business point of view, a diverted ambulance might be thought of as a gurney with a pile of cash on it going to a neighboring/competing hospital. Diversion affects the financial margins of an institution and can make the difference between viability and non-viability. Similarly, when patients are diverted from the operating room because of insufficient operating room times or capacity, margins are affected. The financial incentives for good patient flow are discussed in more detail in the following chapter.

Workforce Stability

As previously stated, patient satisfaction and workforce satisfaction are closely related. In terms of recruiting, training, and acquiring temporary staff, the time and money invested in human resources is enormous, and the benefits of reduced turnover are measurable. More intangible benefits such as employee loyalty and referrals of friends and family as patients and employees also result from a stable workforce.

Regulatory Compliance

Instituting a good flow plan will help administrators meet new regulatory requirements designed to help hospitals create a safer environment at a time when growing demand for services and a shortage of nurses present a challenge. In 2003, the Joint Commission on Accreditation of Healthcare Organizations acknowledged that patient flow is a hospital-wide problem, not just an ED problem (IOM 2006). That acknowledgment is both the good news and the bad news. In the first version of the Joint Commission document, the boarding of patients in the ED was effectively banned. A recent Institute of Medicine (IOM) report supports this and focuses on improving flow. (IOM 2006) Receiving more resistance to that requirement than to any other in its history, the Joint Commission subsequently softened the language and lifted the ban. The commission did, however, enact "flow standards," which mandate that hospitals address system-wide patient flow. According to these standards, a patient may board in the ED only if the care received is comparable to that of an appropriate inpatient ward.

The Joint Commission also now requires that hospitals show that they are developing processes that support efficient patient flow. This accountability is to be folded into the clinical quality improvement process. Further, the commission expects data transparency, with indicators being developed to measure and monitor patient flow. Healthcare organizations are expected to use these measures to improve the flow of patients throughout the system—just one more reason to "get it right."

In addition, the Joint Commission is tracking clinical quality through the use of the so-called "core measures." Since 1986, the Joint Commission has been engaged in a process to develop, test, and implement sets of standardized performance measures in five areas: AMI, congestive heart failure, pneumonia, pregnancy, and surgical infection prevention. These measures have begun to be incorporated into the accreditation process with an eye toward the improvement of safety and quality in healthcare.

Since 2004, hospitals have been required to select three core measure sets from the list and to track certain clinical steps or processes to demonstrate compliance and maintain hospital accreditation. Of these measures, the first three have particular relevance to the ED. The three core measure data sets required for reporting (and most relevant to the practice of emergency medicine) and their target mean data are listed in Figures 2.8, 2.9, and 2.10.

Areas of future core measure implementation include pediatric asthma, pain management, ICU care, and inpatient psychiatric services. While these core measures do not specifically address patient flow, they do relate to the goals of attaining improved flow. With time parameters established for aspects of treatment, such as time to thrombolytics and angioplasty in acute AMI patients, hospital and emergency staff must be able to perform procedures or administer therapies within a brief window of time.

A number of organizations have collaborated with the Joint Commission to bring this process about, including the National Quality Forum, Quality Improvement Organizations, and the Institute of Medicine. Further, the Centers for Medicare & Medicaid Services (CMS) decided in September 2004 to have its quality documentation requirements dovetail with those of the Joint Commission. This collaboration will help control the administrative burdens placed on healthcare institutions. CMS is increasingly moving toward a pay-for-performance model of reimbursement.

While the Joint Commission requirements for flow, standard treatments, and accountability may lead to increased administrative costs for compliance, the outcome will be well worth the price. The partnership between the Joint Commission and hospitals with respect to the commitment to achieve better patient flow creates a climate in which everyone—patients, staff, and administrators—benefits from timely service.

Figure 2.8. Acute Myocardial Infarction Core Measures Goals:
Mean Data Based on Pilot Studies

Aspirin at arrival	94%
ACE Inhibitor for left ventricular systolic dysfunction	83%
Adult smoking cessation counseling	65%
Beta blocker at arrival	85%
Time to thrombolytics	30 minutes
Time to PTCA	90 minutes
Mortality Rate	.09%

Figure 2.9. Heart Failure Core Measures Goals:
Mean Data Based on Pilot Studies

Discharge instructions	28%
Left ventricular function assessment	79%
Ace inhibitors	86%
Smoking cessation counseling	39%

Figure 2.10. Community Acquired Pneumonia Core Measures:
Mean Data Based on Pilot Studies

Oxygen assessment		95%
Pneumococcal vaccine screening		29%
Blood cultures prior to ABs		79%
Smoking cessation counseling:	Adults	35%
	Children	18%
Time to antibiotics		3.2 hours (194 minutes)

Benefits of a Flow Innovation

While one goal of achieving optimal patient flow is to end the practice of boarding, the practice may need to continue while a hospital implements its flow plan. A closer look at one flow strategy reveals the benefits that are possible even when, despite other flow initiatives, the ED becomes overburdened. In the late 1990s, Dr. Peter Viccellio at Stony Brook and Drs. Thom Mayer and Bob Cates at Inova Fairfax Hospital independently began to question the notion that patients could be boarded only in ED hallways. They investigated the supposition that fire regulations made it illegal to board patients in upstairs hallways. It turns out that in most states where this Full Capacity Protocol (Stony Brook) or Adopt-a-Boarder program (Inova) has been implemented, no such prohibitive regulations exist. The teams championed the idea of "sharing the pain" of overcrowding. Rather than having the ED board increasing numbers of patients, they argued that when the ED is boarding and there are no beds for new ED patients, each inpatient unit should in turn be required to board one to two patients. Miraculously, the staff at Stony Brook and Inova went months before a patient actually boarded in the inpatient corridors; a bed was somehow always found.

A completely unexpected positive outcome of this strategy was decreased inpatient length of stay. At a number of sites it was observed that patients boarding in inpatient hallways had almost a full day shorter length of stay (LOS) than patients boarding in the ED. It has been postulated that patients begin getting specialty care earlier on the wards than they do in the ED and thus the LOS is shorter. In fact, at Stony Brook, patients who were boarded in inpatient units had an average LOS of 5.4 days, while the ED boarders had an average LOS of 6.2 days. Facilitated discharges, improved thallium stress-testing turnarounds, inpatient bed expansions, and improved staffing ratios have all been offshoots of the protocol.

The graphs demonstrate the success of the Stony Brook protocol in clinical, fiscal, and patient satisfaction terms. Figure 2.11 shows that when patients were boarded on inpatient wards rather

Figure 2.11. LOS Comparison at Stony Brook

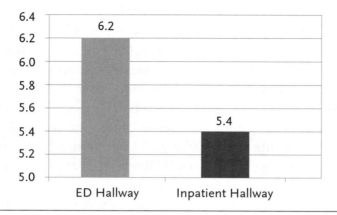

than ED wards, their overall hospital length of stay was decreased by almost a full day. This statistic has significant implications for administrators with regard to the ability to facilitate bed turns. Clinically, from the patient's point of view, this is also good news and suggests that the appropriate care is being given sooner on the wards than in the ED, resulting in faster recovery of the patient. Figure 2.12 shows Press-Ganey scores after the implementation of this protocol. The higher satisfaction score was no surprise to Dr. Viccellio's team, who had surveyed patients and found that they preferred the hospital corridors to the ED corridors.

The Full Capacity Protocol and the Adopt-a-Boarder initiatives have been similarly adapted with great success at other hospitals, including Duke, William Beaumont, Yale, St. Barnabas Health Care System, and Harris Methodist.

Controlling, managing, and facilitating patient flow through the ED and throughout the hospital makes sense to administrators along a variety of parameters. From patient complaints to patient safety, from medical errors to regulatory requirements, from workforce satisfaction to bed turns, taking an aggressive leadership role with respect to patient flow is a win-win proposition. However, improved flow cannot occur without the support and commitment

Figure 2.12. Stony Brook Press–Ganey Patient Satisfaction Survey Results

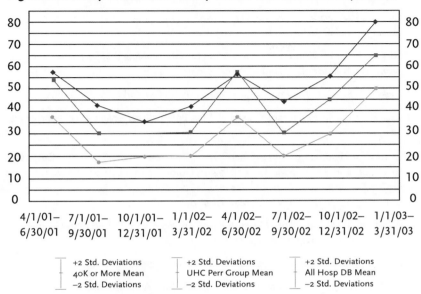

4/1/01–	7/1/01–	10/1/01–	1/1/02–	4/1/02–	7/1/02–	10/1/02–	1/1/03–
6/30/01	9/30/01	12/31/01	3/31/02	6/30/02	9/30/02	12/31/02	3/31/03

+2 Std. Deviations	+2 Std. Deviations	+2 Std. Deviations
40K or More Mean	UHC Perr Group Mean	All Hosp DB Mean
−2 Std. Deviations	−2 Std. Deviations	−2 Std. Deviations

Source: Press-Ganey Report for Stony Brook Hospital. Used with permission

of administration, especially at the highest levels. In other words, it cannot occur without you.

References

Badaracco, J. L., and R. R. Ellsworth. 1989. *Leadership and the Quest for Integrity* Boston: Harvard Business School Press.

Berwick, D. M. 1996. "A Primer on Leading the Improvement of Systems." *British Medical Journal* 312 (7031): 619–22.

BestPractices, Inc. 2005. Anonymous questionnaire of ED nurses at Inova Fairfax Hospital. Fairfax, VA. September.

Boudreaux, E. D., and E. L. O'Hea. 2004. "Patient Satisfaction in the Emergency Department: A Review of the Literature and Implications for Practice." *Journal of Emergency Medicine* 26 (1): 13–26.

Bursch, B., J. Beezy, and R. Shaw. 1993. "Emergency Department Satisfaction: What Matters Most?" *Annals of Emergency Medicine* 22 (3): 586–91.

Cameron, P. A. 2006. "Hospital Overcrowding: A Threat to Patient Safety?" *Medical Journal of Australia.* 184 (5): 203–04

Corrigan, J., and L. Kohn. 2000. To Err Is Human: *Building a Safer Healthcare System.* Washington, DC: National Academies Press.

Drucker, P. F. 1994. *The Practice of Management.* New York: HarperCollins.

Duke, P. 2004. "If ER Nurses Crash. Will Patients Follow?" *Newsweek.* February 2, p.12

Institute for Healthcare Improvement. 2005. "100,000 Lives Campaign Getting Started Kit: Rapid Response Teams How-to Guide." [Online information; retrieved 8/29/06.] www.ihi.org/NR/rdonlyres/6541BE00-00BC-4AD8-A049-CD76EDE5F171/0/RRTHowtoGuidepostedtoweb60806.doc

Institute of Medicine. 2006. *Hospital-Based Emergency Care: At the Breaking Point.* Washington, D. C.: National Academies Press

Kotter, J. 1996. *Leading Change.* Boston: Harvard Business School Press.

Leape, L. L. 1994. "Error in Medicine." *Journal of the American Medical Association* 272 (23): 1851–57.

Maister, D. H. 1985. "The Psychology of Waiting Lines." In *The Service Encounter: Managing Employee/Customer Interaction in Service Business*, edited by J.A. Czepiel et al., 113–23. Lexington, MA: Lexington Books.

McCraig, L. F., and E. W. Nawar. 2006. "National Hospital Ambulatory Medical Care Survey: 2004 Emergency Department Survey." *Advance Data From Vital and Health Statistics* No. 372. National Center for Health Statistics.

Peters, T. 2005. *Tom Peters Essentials: Talent.* London: Dorling Kindersley Publishers Ltd.

Press, I. 2005. *Patient Satisfaction: Defining, Measuring and Improving the Experience of Care.* Chicago: Health Administration Press.

Richardson, D. B. 2006. "Increase in Patient Mortality at 10 Days Associated With Emergency Department Overcrowding. *Medical Journal of Australia.* 184 (5): 213–16

Save Our Emergency Rooms. 2002. "Studies Confirm Gulf Coast Trauma Care System Crisis." [Online press release; retrieved 9/26/06.] http://www.saveourers.org/pr_03.html

Sprivulis, P. C., J. A. Da Silva, I. G. Jacobs, A. R. Frazer, and G. A. Jelinek. 2006. "The Association Between Hospital Overcrowding and Mortality Among Patients

Admitted Via Western Australian Emergency Departments." *Medical Journal of Australia*. 184 (5): 208–12

Further Recomended Readings

Mayer, T. A. and R. Cates. 2004. *Leadership for Great Customer Service*. Chicago: Health Administration Press.

Sobel, D. S. 1995. "Rethinking Medicine: Improving Health Outcomes with Cost-Effective Psychosocial Interventions." *Psychosomatic Medicine* 57 (3): 234–44.

Stony Brook Full Capacity Protocol. Administrative Policies and Procedures. [Online article; retrieved 9/22/05.] www.viccellio.com/fullcapacity.htm.

Sun, B. C., J. Adams, E. J. Orav, D. W. Rucker, T. A. Brennan, and H. R. Burstin. 2000. "Determinants of Patient Satisfaction and Willingness to Return with Emergency Care." *Annals of Emergency Medicine* 35(5): 426–34.

Wilson, M., and K. Nguyen, 2004. "Bursting at the Seams: Improving Patient Flow to Help America's Emergency Departments." Urgent Matters [Online whitepaper; retrieved 9/17/05.] http://www.urgentmatters.org/pdf/UM_WhitePaper_BurstingAtTheSeams.pdf.

Worthington, K. 2004 "Customer Satisfaction in the Emergency Department." *Emergency Medicine Clinics of North America* 22 (1): 87–102.

CHAPTER 3

The Business Case for Patient Flow

You have to do well to do good.

The Institute of Medicine report, Crossing the Quality Chasm (IOM 2001), characterizes quality healthcare as "safe, effective, efficient, timely, patient-centered and equitable." While improving patient flow clearly contributes to all of these aims, does it make sense from a business point of view? You bet it does. In fact, making the financial case for improving flow is fairly simple: Good flow results in increased capacity to provide service, while fixed costs remain the same and variable costs increase only marginally. When a hospital's current costs or financial pressures are considered, the business benefits make their own compelling case for improving patient flow: increased revenue, reduced costs, reduced waste and rework, improved service, improved quality, and improved safety.

First, healthcare is a service business that operates in a climate of distinct competition for attention and resources. Most patients have choices about where to obtain their healthcare. As the baby boomers age, consumer demand for improved service, timeliness, and convenience will rise exponentially. Healthcare systems will have to meet these demands to remain competitive. Innovations to improve patient flow can not only provide the antidote to shrinking margins and loss of market share; they can actually be drivers of improved service and increased financial margins.

NO MARGIN, NO MISSION

The primary mission in healthcare is service to patients and communities. This mission has a critical business component: When service is poor, business decreases. When business is poor, we may be unable to deliver the service to the community that it is our mission to deliver. Therefore, the goal of flow improvement is *both* financial success and quality—not *either* financial success *or* quality. Fortunately, because the two components work symbiotically, the business of healthcare should not conflict with the mission of healthcare—they should be complementary. Good flow means good patient service and quality, as well as a healthy bottom line.

FINANCIAL SUCCESS AND QUALITY
Patient Velocity, Revenue Velocity, and Bed Turns

A simple yet accurate means of understanding the business case for flow comes from the concept of "patient velocity," invented by Thom Mayer and first developed in the ED setting by Best Practices, Inc., but also applicable on the inpatient side. Patient velocity is a simple ratio of billable patient visits divided by the number of hours of clinical coverage required to effectively evaluate and treat such patients.

$$\text{Patient Velocity} = \frac{\text{number of patients}}{\text{number of hours of clinical coverage}}$$

At its simplest level, the numerator (number of patients) translates to revenues, while the denominator (number of hours of clinical coverage) translates to costs, in this case the labor costs to treat the patients. Thus, in the ED setting, as flow initiatives increase the ability to see more patients, profitability increases as functional capacity grows. In a typical ED setting, effective flow initiatives can improve patient velocity from 1.6 or 1.7 patients per hour to greater than 2.0 patients per hour, which drives substantial profitability for both the hospital and the physician group.

The same metric applies on the inpatient side with regard to bed turns, or revenues versus costs per case-adjusted admissions. As flow initiatives improve capacity, patient velocity or bed turns also improve. Think in terms of the life cycle of one patient bed over the course of a year. How many times per year is that bed turned to serve another inpatient? The more bed turns per year (a flow metric), the more revenue per bed. Fixed costs remain stable; marginal costs are low.

Let's take this a step further. Let's pretend that you are the owner of the Cheesecake Factory. In terms of service and profitability, which metric are you more interested in—the number of tables occupied at noon (the equivalent of the midnight census) or the number of times that table is turned over for new customers during peak periods? The answer is obvious: all things staying the same (food quality, customer satisfaction, staff satisfaction), it is table turns that matter. On the inpatient side, this concept has been pioneered by the IHI.

As will be discussed in Chapter 6, an effective hospitalist program can reduce inpatient length of stay by 1.5 to 2.5 days, largely through the use of treatment protocols and early discharge plans. This program, therefore, creates additional bed capacity through quicker bed turns or improved patient velocity, while at the same time having a significant financial impact because fixed costs remain the same.

A final aspect of the financial formulas for flow is the concept of "revenue velocity." Revenue velocity in the ED is simply patient velocity times the net collected revenue per patient:

Billable patients (revenue)

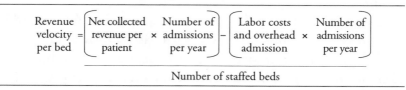

$$\text{Revenue velocity} = \frac{\text{Revenue per provider hour}}{} = \left(\frac{\text{Patients per hour}}{} \times \frac{\text{Hours of coverage}}{} \times \frac{\text{Net collected revenue per patient}}{}\right) - \left(\frac{\text{Hours of coverage}}{} \times \frac{\text{Cost per provider hour}}{}\right)$$

On the inpatient side, the formula is as follows:

Billable patient admissions

$$\text{Revenue velocity per bed} = \frac{\left(\frac{\text{Net collected revenue per patient}}{} \times \frac{\text{Number of admissions per year}}{}\right) - \left(\frac{\text{Labor costs and overhead}}{} \times \frac{\text{Number of admissions per year}}{}\right)}{\text{Number of staffed beds}}$$

The same concept can be applied to any unit for which profitability as a function of service velocity is desired. Using this simple formula, we can clearly see that flow efforts improve capacity, which in turn increases patient velocity and, therefore, profitability increases.

Is it possible to be too fast? In other words, can patient velocity and/or bed turns be pushed too far—to the point that increasing profitability has a negative impact on other indicators, including patient satisfaction, quality measures, patient safety, and risk reduction? Absolutely. For this reason, patient velocity should be balanced against other aspects of care, preferably in a measured and formal fashion. Balancing measures are critical.

"That which cannot be measured cannot be improved" (W. Edwards Deming). In an effort to measure the interplay of finances, flow, and the other aspects of care, Thom Mayer, Kirk Jensen, Rick Torres and BestPractices, Inc., have developed a balanced dashboard approach known as the 4-S Dashboard™, comprising elements of science/safety (clinical protocols/risk reductions), service (patient satisfaction), sustainability (financial measures), and superior leadership (Figure 3.1).

While the dashboard is a graphic indicator of the interplay of financial and other forces that comprise flow, other perspectives on financial feasibility are useful as well.

Figure 3.1. The 4-S Dashboard™

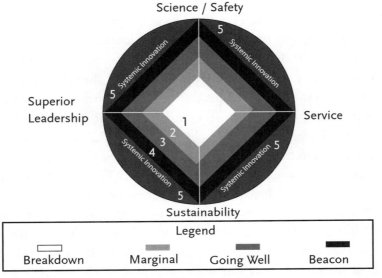

Sheila Leatherman and colleagues, in *The Business Case for Quality Case Studies and Analysis* (Leatherman et al. 2003), explains the method for determining whether an innovation is financially viable:

> A business case for a health care improvement intervention exists if the entity that invests in the intervention realizes a financial return on its investment in a reasonable time frame, using a reasonable rate of discounting. This may be realized as *"bankable dollars"* (profit), a reduction in losses for a given program or population, or avoided costs. In addition, a *business case* may exist if the investing entity believes that a positive indirect effect on organizational function and sustainability will accrue within a reasonable time frame.

In short, a business case exists if a program results in more profit, reduces losses, or avoids potential costs (such as those inherent in too-high overhead or in rework).

INCREASING VOLUME

One way to increase profit is to serve more customers. With good flow, your healthcare system can serve more people with the same staff and serve them well. Bed turns can be increased, while maintaining the focus on quality service. Simply moving people through the system quickly is not the goal. Consider the financial implications—calculate the opportunity cost per day, per month, or per year. What would happen if you increased admissions by 5 percent? That is the return on investment. From another angle, consider the ED revenue potential for a one-hour throughput reduction. If your ED has 40,000 visits per year at an average of three to four hours per patient visit and you reduce the average length of stay by one hour, this results in a potential 400,000 hours of increased service capacity. This can allow for an additional 10,000 to 13,000 patient visits. If you multiply 10,000 new patient visits by $500 in outpatient revenue for each visit, *the result is an impressive $5 million potential revenue increase. This does not include the increase in inpatient revenue from ED admissions.* On the inpatient side, figure anywhere from $5,000 to $8,000 in profit (on average) and multiply that by the number of increased admissions per year. The numbers are staggering.

If the commitment to patient flow and service is fulfilled, another benefit accrues from reduced throughput time: Patients are more satisfied with the shorter stay and higher quality service. Improved patient satisfaction results in increased "same-store sales." From a financial standpoint, a patient has much more than just a single-visit value. Think in terms of the lifetime value of a patient or healthcare customer.

When determining how improved flow can financially benefit your healthcare system, the following key measures matter in the ED:

- patient volume;
- the number of emergency beds and bed turns;
- staffing hours per patient;
- ED LOS or cycle time; and
- patient satisfaction with services.

Equivalent measures on the inpatient side are as follows:

- patient volume;
- the number of functional inpatient beds and bed turns (that is, how many patients a bed services per unit of time);
- staffing hours per admission or per patient;
- LOS; and
- patient satisfaction with services.

Equivalent metrics can be looked at for any unit or microsystem (e.g., surgery, the ICU, telemetry).

When looking at admissions, examine the contribution that each of the incoming patient streams makes to the hospital census. EDs typically contribute from 30 to 70 percent of admissions (with a median of about 50 percent). Surgical admissions generally make up 40 percent of the total number of hospital admissions.

Knowing the admission percentage and the revenue per admission allows a hospital to calculate the revenue per year flowing in from each of the admission sources.

Reducing throughput time increases the efficiency and effectiveness of the staff. It increases the capacity of the emergency, surgical, or inpatient unit or department. It improves staff satisfaction. It improves patient satisfaction and patient outcomes, and it saves money and generates new revenue.

To determine how improving flow can improve profit, ask the following questions: What is the revenue per patient? What is the true cost per patient? What is the revenue generated per ED bed, surgical suite, or inpatient bed, per day, per month, or per year? Monitor admission cycle times, diversion hours, the boarding burden in the ED, PACU, or wherever patients are being held or bottlenecked. Look at the patients who end up not being completely served—the number of ED walk-aways and surgical patients who cannot be scheduled or who have their cases cancelled. With your numbers in hand, you can ask several key questions to determine where revenue can be generated:

1. Is there an unmet demand for services?
2. Is there underutilization of beds or bed turns?
3. Is there underutilization of providers?

If the answer is "yes" to any of the questions above, then improved patient flow can lead to increased service capacity, which leads to increased ED revenue, which leads to increased hospital revenue.

As you examine your own system, be alert for other flow problems that might be limiting capacity. For example, at St. John's Regional Health Center in Springfield, Missouri, a busy trauma center, the operating rooms were so backed up that surgical teams often worked "late at night or into the wee hours of the morning" to keep up with the cases. Examining their data, Christina Dempsey (2004), vice president for perioperative services, noted an interesting fact: The unscheduled surgeries, those coming in from the ED, occurred in regular and predictable numbers. However, because they were never planned for, these unscheduled surgeries delayed the regularly scheduled surgeries, often pushing these procedures into the middle of the night. By making a radical change and setting aside one of the 22 operating rooms for unscheduled cases and somewhat altering block scheduling, the hospital smoothed its flow, eliminated the late-night schedule, and unexpectedly increased its revenue. Rather than limiting capacity, the new plan brought a 5 percent increase in surgical case volume and a 4.6 percent revenue increase. Everybody was happy, especially the surgeons who had frequently been working at 3 a.m.

REDUCING LOSSES

The Cost of Boarding

In many clinical situations, beds are the rate-limiting factor. Therefore, if the culture of your healthcare system supports the boarding of admitted patients in the ED, this practice is costing you money. The

Figure 3.2. Discrete Opportunity Costs

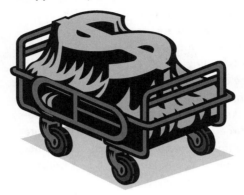

Source: Getty Images, Inc. Used with permission.

boarding burden significantly impacts your ED service capacity, with inpatients parked in outpatient beds. This practice impedes financial flow in two distinct ways: It blocks ED service capacity and it limits the number of bed turns upstairs. It also overextends ED staff, creating a chaotic environment for both the healthcare team and patients. These factors, in turn, cost the system in terms of higher risk of medical error, service lapses, and dissatisfied patients.

The Cost of Diversion

Hospital diversions are the patients the ED does not have capacity to see and are therefore sent to another facility. A discrete opportunity cost exists for every patient diverted (Figure 3.2). Some hospitals have estimated this cost to be as high as $300 per hour of diversion or as high as $7,000 to $8,000 for each diverted admission. If one admission generates $7,000 to $8,000 in profit, then the number of diverted patients per month or per year times the net revenue per patient equals the opportunity cost of diverting patients. You should do the math for your own facility.

Figure 3.3. The Cost of a Complaint

Physician time for record review and follow-up with patient	1 hour	$100
Medical director time for record review	30 minutes	$50
Medical records pulling charts, copying	30 minutes	$8
Business office copying bills, explanation, rebilling	30 minutes	$20
Secretary checking ED charges	15 minutes	$10
ED manager time	30 minutes	$30
Administrative time to review (if needed)	30 minutes	$35
Patient relations initial complaint, investigation, referral, follow-up	2 hours	$40
Supplies	30 minutes	$10
Bill adjustments		$100
TOTAL:		$400

The cost of transfers due to limited inpatient capacity is calculated similarly. A hypothetical scenario: If the hospital transfers 23 patients per month, the revenue loss, a value of $1,178 per patient day times four days, totals approximately $1,600,000 per year.

The Cost of Patient Complaints

While the technical quality in healthcare is unparalleled, service quality often leaves much to be desired. Patients interpret the quality of the service as a function of how well things work (operations management). Even if a patient's medical problem is treated adequately, or even more than adequately, a long wait or poor treatment by the frontline provider may leave the patient dissatisfied with her care. Let's take another look at the systemic costs of poor service or poor quality. Chuck Chakrapani (1998) divides these costs into two categories: visible and invisible. The visible costs of poor quality are the cost of handling irate customers, the cost of losing customers, and the cost of rework. The invisible costs of poor quality are the cost of countering

Figure 3.4. The True Cost of a Patient Complaint

- Each disappointed patient who complains represents six others who are unhappy with a similar experience;
- Therefore each complaint represents seven unhappy patients.
- Each unhappy patient tells eight to ten other people about his unhappy experience;
- 63 people now know about these unhappy experiences.
- One fourth of these 63 people (16) will act on what they hear and will choose not to do business with you.
- 16 patients x average revenue/patient x number of visits/patient/ lifetime = lost revenue per type of complaint.
- 16 patients x $500/patient x 5 lifetime visits = $40,000.
- Just to handle the average complaint costs an institution $400 (or $20,000 per year).
- If 5 percent of inpatients opt not to return each year, the revenue at risk is $2,500,000 per year.
- 95 percent of customers will be satisfied, surprised, and tell others if the problem is resolved on the spot.
- 96 percent of dissatisfied customers never complain.
- It is six times more expensive to attract a new patient than it is to keep an existing one.

negative publicity, the cost of replacing lost customers, and higher marketing costs.

Dissatisfied patients cost a healthcare system in three ways: (1) the financial outlay to manage each complaint, (2) the impact of every unhappy patient on other people who might use your services, and (3) the lifetime value of a patient. Factoring in physician time for record review, medical director time, medical records retrieval and review, business office attention, and management time, writing off a single complaint costs about $400 to $500 (Figure 3.3). Handling dissatisfied patients also frequently involves the time of senior personnel, time that could be put to better use elsewhere.

Figure 3.4 shows that the true cost of a complaint extends far beyond the amount shown in Figure 3.3. Every disappointed patient who complains represents six others who are also unhappy about a similar experience but have not complained. Therefore, every complaint represents seven unhappy patients. The typical dissatisfied patient will tell eight to ten other people. If you have seven dissatisfied patients each telling nine other people or potential patients about their visit, you now have 63 people who know about this unhappy experience. One quarter of these patients (16 out of the 63) will act on what they hear. This means that 16 people are likely not to do business with your hospital or your ED because of this experience of poor service. Multiply these 16 patients by the true profit of each patient visit and you get the approximate cost of each service lapse, not to mention the lifetime value loss for each of these patients. Multiply the lost profit per visit by the number of visits over a patient's lifetime and you can see how much a dissatisfied patient really costs. Assuming an average patient revenue of $5,000 to $8,000 per admission and an average of 10,000 admissions per year, if only 5 percent of dissatisfied patients will not return, the revenue at risk ranges between $2,500,000 and $4,500,000 per year, largely representing pure profit.

Another dissatisfied patient, the one who leaves without being seen by the physician or provider (LWBS), is the embodiment of the missed opportunity—the revenue that goes to another hospital when an ED is on diversion. The LWBSs are patients who arrive at the hospital seeking care and then decide to leave because of waits and delays. The number of these patients who walk away, as well as the number of LBTCs (leave before treatment is complete) and AMAs (leave against medical advice), is often a barometer of the service level and capacity of an ED and certainly reflects turnaround time. Since it is six times more expensive to attract a new customer than to keep an old one, and the easiest patients (customers) to keep are the ones you already have, the patients who leave before treatment represent a revenue loss far beyond the simple cost of the visit (Chapkraponi 1998).

Good patient flow incorporates service that is built into the process and not viewed as an add-on reserved for certain times or certain patients. The result is decreased complaints and increased outpatient and inpatient volume based on customer choice.

COST AVOIDANCE

Medical Error

We have already explored the importance of reduced medical error from a patient safety perspective. From the financial standpoint, improved patient safety and clinical quality are no less critical. Good flow can help an organization avoid the tremendous liability suffered as the result of a medical mishap. The cost of a settlement is exacerbated by the stress on administrators and staff and the damage to the healthcare system's reputation.

System Inefficiencies and Rework

Good patient flow can also help a healthcare system avoid the costs associated with system inefficiencies. When LOS is decreased, for example, resource usage decreases as well. Avoiding backups and overcrowding reduces the increased costs associated with complications arising from poor quality or delays when staff are overextended and exhausted. Reduction of costs is also introduced through the inefficiencies inherent in substandard or slow work—the cost of rework, waste, and resource consumption.

HUMAN RESOURCES

As previously stated, a clear connection exists between patient satisfaction and workforce satisfaction and stability. A stable and satisfied workforce pays off in a variety of ways, some of which may not at first be obvious. The costs of temporary and agency staffing, recruiting, hiring, and training are enormous in a high-turnover system. The cost of replacing an employee is usually estimated to be one-third of his annual wages. Indirect costs include the initial lower productivity and capacity of the new employee. The costs of replacing human capital are exacerbated by attendant missed opportunities for revenue caused by insufficient staff. Consider a few of the hidden costs of an unstable workforce:

- ED diversions and patient transfers from underserved or understaffed areas of the hospital;
- increased waits for surgery; and
- lost productivity and ineffective team building.

Good flow can save human resource money as well. Healthcare systems with good flow attract good workers, who may then recommend the workplace to other job seekers—friends, neighbors, and family members. Creating a magnet workplace can give a healthcare system a tremendous advantage in hiring and retaining nurses, for example. When the cost of turnover is quantified, good flow makes sound financial sense and provides a competitive advantage in the marketplace that positions the system to achieve a solid return on investment.

MAKING THE BUSINESS CASE FOR IMPROVING PATIENT FLOW

Show me the money.
—From the movie *Jerry McGuire*

From a business perspective, the most important hospital indicators are financial performance, patient satisfaction, and the reputation of the healthcare system. "Hard green dollars" come from operational performance enhancement, ED crowding solutions, diversion management, optimizing surgical flow, and increased admissions. These dollars are spent on wages, equipment, operations, maintenance, supplies, medication, and so on. Hard green dollars disappear when patients are lost due to diversion, as walkaways, or from cancelled surgeries. On the other hand, "soft green dollars" come from workforce satisfaction, patient satisfaction, medical staff satisfaction, and hospital board satisfaction. How do we connect the flow improvement effort to the hard and soft green dollars? Simple: Changes to improve flow lead to improved performance, which leads to decreased costs and increased revenue, and thus greater profit.

To persuade your healthcare system to commit to a plan for improving flow, you must make the connection between flow and both soft and hard green dollars. Progress toward a higher quality of care often hinges on the strength of the business case for patient flow. If the business case is not convincingly linked to the flow improvement efforts, senior management may undervalue the initiative and fail to give it sufficient priority and support. Because senior executive involvement is critical, financial incentives should be clarified and aligned. There must be clear-cut goals for success and quality that involve speed, service, and a fair cost. A business plan should include a statement of product or services, cost assumptions, revenue assumptions, a cash flow statement, a sensitivity analysis, a risk analysis, a work plan, and roll-out strategies. Identifying and publicizing examples of how or where improved patient flow has led to direct improvements in the bottom line can be critical in the early phases of the initiative.

Where are the opportunities for improvement? The opportunities exist in taking a leadership approach that involves quality control and quality improvement and incorporating it into the design, production, and operations of the healthcare system. Healthcare is a labor-intensive industry in which customers are treated one patient at a time. The challenge is to reduce costs while also improving quality. This can be done by undertaking the following:

- aligning incentives;
- redesigning the system;
- matching capacity and demand;
- attending to the finances;

- reducing cycle times;
- eliminating non-value-added steps in processes; and
- reducing unnecessary work.

The goal is to improve quality and throughput and to link this improvement to the financial results.

Throughout this book we encourage the development of pilot projects with specific goals, measures, and outcomes. The plan-do-study-act methodology of testing changes (see more in Chapter 5) is really a variation of the scientific method: Observe, formulate a hypothesis (predict), experiment (test the hypothesis), and then reevaluate. The results of these efforts need to be incorporated into the healthcare system's financial scorecard or dashboard, and the financial impact of these programs needs to be measured and publicized. Publication of results can contribute to the establishment of a uniform system to measure clinical and customer service performance. Such a system offers tremendous opportunities to reduce waste and improve quality throughout the healthcare community.

Making the business case can reinvigorate our efforts to work on improving patient flow, yet we need to take a balanced scorecard approach to the business case. It isn't just about the money. It isn't just about the business. In our increasingly complex healthcare systems, the connection between quality and reimbursement has often been lost, and financial incentives have often been misaligned. With good flow, the return on investment from improvements in operations management are potentially significant, as are the benefits for patients and the healthcare workforce. Financial margins are important, but so are clinical and operational quality and customer and workforce satisfaction. With good flow design, you don't have to choose between these goals.

References

Chakrapani, C. 1998. *How to Measure Service Quality and Customer Satisfaction.* Chicago: American Marketing Association.

Dempsey, C., and K. Larson. 2004. "Can't we all just get along?: Know your role in fostering hospital-provider collaboration." *Nursing Management.* 35 (11): 32–35

Institute of Medicine. 2001. *Crossing the Quality Chasm: A New Health System for the 21st Century.* Washington, DC: National Academies Press.

Leatherman, S., D. Berwick, D. Iles, L. S. Lewin, F. Davidoff, T. Nolan, and M. Bisognano. 2003. "The Business Case for Quality: Case Studies and an Analysis." *Health Affairs (Millwood)* 22 (2): 17–30.

Further Recommended Readings

Beckwith, H. 1997. *Selling the Invisible: A Field Guide to Modern Marketing.* New York: Warner Books, Inc.

Berwick, D. M., A. B. Godfrey, and J. Roessner. 1990. *Curing Health Care: New Strategies for Quality Improvement.* San Francisco: Jossey-Bass.

Cleverley, W. O., and A. E. Cameron. 2003. *Essentials of Health Care Finance.* Sudbury, MA: Jones and Bartlett Publishers.

Customer Service: Tips for Taking the Best Care of Customers. Economic Press, No 352.

Evans, C. J. 2000. *Financial Feasibility Studies for Healthcare.* New York: McGraw-Hill.

Fahrney, P. 1999. *Benchmark Standards in the ED–Part 2, Continuous Quality Improvement.*

Fitzsimmons, J., and M. Fitzsimmons. 2006. *Service Management: Operations, Strategy, Information Technology.* 5th ed. Boston: McGraw-Hill.

Stahl, M. J., and P. J. Dean. 1999. *The Physician's Essential MBA: What Every Physician Leader Needs to Know.* Gaithersburg, MD: Aspen Publishers.

Zelman, W. N., M. J. McCue, and A.R. Millikan. 1999. *Financial Management of Healthcare Organizations.* Malden, MA: Blackwell Publishing.

CHAPTER 4

Leadership for Patient Flow

Managers do things right. Leaders do the right things.
—Warren Bennis, *On Becoming a Leader*

PERHAPS THE BEDROCK principle of flow is that it requires strong, effective, and persistent leadership; good management, good measurements, and good intentions are simply not enough. What is leadership? It's a popular subject—an Internet search of the word results in over 8,000 books and articles on the subject, so a comprehensive review is beyond our scope here. Instead, let's listen to some of the best voices on leadership, particularly those on leading change, since effective flow requires a fundamental cultural change focused on removing barriers to flow. The patient must be at the center of the healthcare experience. Just as we looked through a series of lenses to focus on flow, we'll do the same here, with leadership in our sights.

Warren Bennis's (2003) point about the difference between leadership and management is essential: It is not enough to be efficient—efficiency must be in service of the right direction. Leadership sets that direction and continues to adjust the course over time. The authors' extensive experience coaching and mentoring flow initiatives has shown us that effective flow requires fundamental change within the organization, which simply cannot occur without leadership. Systems thinker Russell Ackoff (1981) has noted that second-order change represents changes *within* an organization, while first-order change involves changes *of* an organization. Flow requires first-order change, and therefore effective leadership.

John Kotter (2002) of Harvard Business School has tremendous insight into the relationship between leadership and management:

> Leadership works through people and culture. It's soft and hot. Management works through hierarchy and systems. It's harder and cooler. The fundamental purpose of management is to keep the current system functioning. The fundamental purpose of leadership is to produce change, especially non-incremental change.

So which set of skills is needed to maximize flow—leadership or management? It is easy to see that flow requires change—indeed, even "non-incremental change"—which points us toward leadership as an essential set of skills that are fundamental to flow. Without question, flow requires leadership.

Nonetheless, the more subtle point is that, in the midst of change, we have to keep the elements of the system that have not directly been changed functioning. That requires management skills. So here's the question: Do I need leadership or management skills to improve flow in my healthcare system? The answer is, "Yes!" You need both sets of skills to succeed at improving flow. (See Peter Block's wonderful book *The Answer to "How" Is "Yes"* [2001] for more on this.) Keep in mind Kotter's (2002) trenchant observation: "Most companies are over-managed and under-led."

COMMITMENT TO FLOW

With the benefits of good flow clearly defined and with the wisdom of leadership gurus in hand, how can you begin to lead change? Here we offer a set of key principles and ideas that you can use to get started. We will later explore the theories and methods for improving flow. For patient flow efforts to be successful, you and your leadership team must have a deep desire to put these principles and methods to the test. Experience shows us that teams, departments, and hospitals often get bogged down in the quest for ideas, at the expense of taking action. Principles and ideas are necessary, but they are not sufficient. What is really needed is unshakable commitment by high-level senior administrators and an absolute focus on and dedication to execution. To create change in flow, performance must be sustained over time. Change in flow is not an effort that can be undertaken over several months or several quarters. A sustained and unrelenting effort will be required for as long as one to two years to create a largely self-sustaining chain reaction.

Leadership commitment must be visible. Get out on the "shop floor." Go down into the ED when it is busy, and walk the route that a patient would take. Look at the waiting room. Is it clean? Is it friendly? Is it conducive to good patient care? Are patients being acknowledged as they arrive? How is the greeter or service person behaving? Is he keeping patients and families informed? How are people being treated? What are they doing while they wait? What is it like to walk into the clinical care area? The ED team may be busy, but are they focused on patient care or frustrated because of poor patient flow and subpar clinical processes? Talk to some of the patients waiting to be treated and talk to some of the patients that *have* been treated to get a sense of what their experience is like. Talk to the physicians and nursing staff. Do they feel fulfilled in their work? Do they have a sense that they are accomplishing their mission? Repeat this activity on all your units and floors, both when things are quiet and when things are busy. Making yourself available and your commitment to positive change visible to the organization demonstrates your commitment to and passion for improving the experience for both patients and staff.

THREE STEPS IN CHANGE

Kurt Lewin, in *Resolving Social Conflicts* (1948), has noted three major steps in the process of change:

1. unfreezing, or shocking the system out of stasis;
2. transforming, or making purposeful adjustments; and
3. refreezing, or ingraining adjustments into the system.

Consider the following simple example.

> The Patient Flow Team at Inova Fairfax Hospital used performance improvement data to show that a bolus effect of four to six patients typically presented to the triage area at approximately 8:30 a.m. to 10 a.m. on most days. These patients were triaged, one by one, and sent to room assignments, one by one. This process caused unnecessary delays, as the flow team pointed out, since these patients would be seen by the same nurses, technicians, and doctors, using the same rooms. How to improve *flow?*
>
> *Unfreezing:* The Patient Flow Team used data to show that the arrival times, acuity, and unused capacity (rooms available in the ED) were highly predictable. Therefore, the team suggested "unfreezing," or changing, the old rule (triage one at a time) that had been followed for decades.
>
> *Transforming:* The team considered the old rule an obstacle that stood in the way of flow and brainstormed with doctors, nurses, ED technicians, and registration to uncover ideas about how this process could change. The ED nurses, who would be most affected by the transformation, suggested a new rule: "direct to room." This rule stated that when a queue formed at triage at times when rooms were available in the ED treatment area, patients would be sent directly to the rooms, where triage and bedside registration would be performed.
>
> *Refreezing:* After considerable discussion and refinement by the ED team members, direct to room was established as a formal policy of the ED at Inova Fairfax Hospital. Internal cycle data

consistently showed that this flow initiative reduced ED turn-around time by nearly 30 minutes for these patients. Thus, the new rule was established as the new standard in the organization after rapid cycle testing (discussed in more detail in Chapter 5), which verified its positive effect on flow.

As the terms "unfreezing," "transforming," and "refreezing" suggest, creating change is a dynamic process. To create change in flow, you must improve or transform performance over time.

LEADERSHIP STYLE

For years, researchers at the University of Rhode Island have worked with a compelling change model that focuses on the personal perspective on change. This model has the following five steps:

1. *Precontemplation* is when there is no desire to change.
2. *Contemplation* is when there is a desire to change, but nothing is being done.
3. *Preparation* is when initial steps are undertaken for change.
4. *Action* is when steps are actually taken.
5. *Maintenance* is maintaining or holding the gains.

As the Rhode Island model so aptly illustrates, change is not an event but a process that engages human behavior. Leaders must establish will, optimism, trust, and urgency, focusing on steps 3, 4, and 5. Both leadership and management skills are essential to engage the team and to be successful. Jim Collins, in *Good to Great* (2001), notes the importance of what he calls "Level 5" leaders, people more like Abraham Lincoln and Socrates than George Patton or Julius Caesar. Level 5 leaders combine personal humility and professional will.

Level 5 leaders are ambitious, but their ambition is first and foremost for the institution, not for themselves. This model of dedication to the success of the enterprise as a collective achievement works well for leading change to improve patient flow. Great military commanders like Patton and Caesar, while highly effective in battle, typically lack the humility to subordinate their role within the far more expansive goals of the institution. What Level 5 leaders know is that successful leadership requires the courage to encourage (literally to give courage to those you lead) others to think and act in new and evolutionary, if not revolutionary, ways.

> The dogmas of the quiet past are inadequate to the stormy present. The occasion is piled high with difficulty, and we must rise to the occasion. As our case is new, so we must think anew and act anew. We must disenthrall ourselves, and then we shall save our country!
>
> —Abraham Lincoln

While the situation of improving patient flow may not be as dramatic as that faced by Lincoln, is there a single healthcare leader who doesn't feel called "to the ramparts" to lead our healthcare systems more effectively—and therefore creatively?

The importance of humility in great leaders is underscored by an example from World War II. Steven Ambrose's book *Band of Brothers* (2001) (later popularized in movie form by Tom Hanks and Steven Spielberg) focused on the leadership of Major Dick Winters, who led the 2nd Battalion of the 506th Parachute Infantry Regiment of the 101st Airborne (Screaming Eagles). Here are his terse and compelling reflections:

> Not one man walks around wearing his wings or medals on his chest to stand out. It is what each man carries in his chest that makes him different. It is the confidence, pride and character that makes the WWII generation stand out in any crowd.

The value of humility cannot be stated better.

KEY STRATEGIES FOR LEADING CHANGE

Fortunately, you don't have to be a Lincoln or a Socrates to lead the flow improvement initiative in your hospital. You and your patient flow team, however, will use key strategies to bring about improvements in flow, including the following:

- accept that flow is a complex, technical problem;
- break through the boundaries of multiple departments;
- implement team-developed and team-led flow initiatives (resist the urge to install, layer on, or mandate—simplify and improve whenever possible);
- effectively diagnose the problems, then test your changes;
- change your culture and your processes.

Accept That Flow Is a Complex Technical Problem

From the beginning, leadership requires commitment to solving often thorny logistical problems and to unfreezing rules and processes to which patients and care providers are accustomed. Patients flow into a hospital via the ED, surgical, elective, and direct admit streams. Within the system, they interact with multiple service providers. Many variables—some controllable, some uncontrollable—affect the outcome of the healthcare experience. As presented in the first chapter, solving a problem in one area of the healthcare system may create a problem in another: for example, faster throughput in the ED may overload the ICU; staggered discharge times may result in changes in housekeeping staff hours; changes in operating room scheduling will change physician practices. Achieving improved flow offers an exciting and ongoing challenge—a journey rather than a destination. Not everyone will understand where you are going. Not everyone will be happy with where you are going. Not everyone will be capable of going where you are going.

Break Through the Boundaries of Multiple Departments

Leading change, you will have to break down the walls that divide the separate service providers in your healthcare system and enable people to see beyond their own silos.

> An old dirt farmer who had worked the same small farm his whole life traveled to a big farm meeting where he saw farmers from all over the country. As he sat on a bench outside the meeting center, a cocky young Midwestern farmer came up and asked, "How many acres you farming?" The old farmer said proudly, "I've got 28 of the prettiest acres you ever saw. How 'bout you, son?" The farmer replied, "Well, if I get in my truck at six in the morning, I ain't halfway across my spread at lunchtime." The old farmer said sympathetically, "Shoot, I used to have a truck like that."

Like the old farmer, we all get used to the systems in which we work and often cannot see outside the reality of those systems. Because of the intense nature of the work and the specific skills required, healthcare teams and workers generally lack a broad perspective, working instead only within their own microsystems. Good people attempt to optimize patient care and patient flow within these subsystems, without an understanding or an awareness of what goes on in other parts of the hospital (the whole system). For many, healthcare has always been this way. The goal has been to get through the crises of the day rather than to solve problems at the system level. In traditional hospital structures, individual department leaders often look out for their units in a protective and proprietary way, blocking admissions from overcrowded EDs or PACUs.

Smoothing or optimizing flow at the healthcare system level offers opportunities to permanently change the way hospital microsystems work together. The Adopt-a-Boarder program and Full Capacity Protocol are whole-system responses to this flow-impeding structure. Having available patient care beds (or capacity) on the inpatient side is certainly preferable to having patients in hallways, but these approaches do illustrate the principle of load leveling and a shared-systems response to a flow dilemma in another unit of the hospital.

Solving flow problems requires high levels of cooperation and integration across multiple departments. Flow crosses many boundaries within the hospital and involves many staff members and services. A single discharge, for example, may involve physicians, nurses, lab and radiology technicians, dietitians, pharmacists, business office personnel, transportation schedulers, and volunteers. The gaps that exist between the departments that provide these services must be bridged, establishing effective organization and communication. Structuring the flow team to include leaders from all areas of the healthcare system helps make this happen. So do position exchanges (letting employees see what it is like to work in another department) and rewards for innovative flow solutions. When the gaps are bridged, the wins can be tremendous for patients, staff, and leaders.

For example, simply encouraging communication between hospital departments or units can lead to welcome surprises. At one hospital, when the lab manager was brought onto the flow team, a simple discussion of turnaround time for lab tests led to significant time savings:

Flow team: "We would like to get our tests back faster from the lab."

Lab manager: "Well, I do have a new centrifuge that could save you 25 minutes on several key lab tests—that won't help much, will it?"

Flow team: "Won't help! When can you get it!?"

Lab manager: "Tomorrow—we didn't know 25 minutes would help you."

While the 25 minutes seemed insignificant to the lab, it was a lifetime to the ED doctor, nurse, or patient. What if every test came back 25 minutes faster? The opportunity for one provider to know how his service affected another created real improvement in the system. Add up those saved minutes on all ED tests sent to the lab in a day—in a week, in a month, in a year—to get the true impact of one simple team interaction and process change. Everybody wins—the patients and the people who take care of those patients.

Breaking down the silos does involve changing the organizational culture (discussed in more detail later) and, like most changes to improve flow, requires buy-in at the highest levels of administration. Though frontline change works best from the bottom up with patient care teams, it cannot occur without an ideology that is iterated from the top down and supported in every way.

Implement Team-Developed and Team-Led Flow Initiatives

Medical care today is a team sport, so a full team, the right team, an experienced team, a harmonious team, is necessary. You want to field your best team—your A-team members—who are positive, proactive, and compassionate. You do not want B-team members who are negative, reactive, or confused. Teamwork should be woven into the fabric of your culture and your approach to patient care. Teamwork can be taught, improved, and sustained through a commitment to excellent service, communication, and long-term relationships with colleagues and essential (ancillary) partners.

The management of people is at the root of most improvement project problems, and as a result many of these issues can be resolved with effective people management. Dwight Eisenhower, as military commander of the Allied Expeditionary Force in World War II, aptly summarized the change leader's challenge: "My experience is that leadership requires the ability to get people to go where they do not want to go—while making them think it was their idea in the first place."

Figure 4.1. Maslow's Hierarchy of Needs

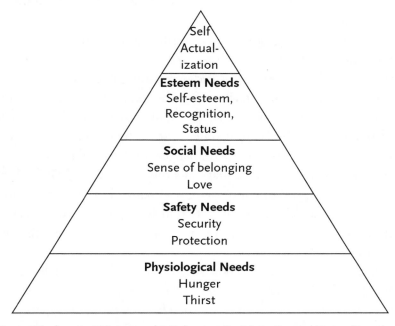

Source: Maslow, A., R. Frager, and J. Fadman. 1987. *Motivation and Personality,* 3rd edition. Adapted by permission of Pearson Education, Inc., Upper Saddle River, NJ.

As a leader of change, you must empower an A-team of change leaders to determine what needs to be done and to implement the changes. In establishing the structure and facilitating change, you must be prepared to understand and overcome employee resistance, anxiety, and even anger. When change threatens the status quo, people often resist, even if the change will ultimately improve working conditions and quality of service. People fear change and the unknown. At the most basic level, they may be worried about their performance and their jobs. They wonder where they will fit into the new way of doing things, how they will adapt to new expectations, and how they will be evaluated. Maslow's hierarchy of needs places human physiologic and safety needs at the bottom, while esteem and self-actualization needs are at the top (Figure 4.1). To understand these needs and to lead people through a process when their security is threatened, a little empathy and a great deal of communication and encouragement go a long way.

Furthermore, we are often comfortable with our current processes and don't think about ways to improve patient flow throughout the entire system. People working in the system think, "If it ain't broke, don't fix it," or, "The devil you know is better than the devil you don't." It is very hard to see a future state that is different from the current state, even if the current state is less than ideal. The temptation is to just get through today, or to keep your head down and think that "this too shall pass." This is often the response, too, if previous plans for change in the organization have lacked sufficient will or were poorly implemented. The staff think, "Why bother to adapt to another 'here today, gone tomorrow' directive?"

Sometimes, resistance takes the form of criticism or hostility. Most people are better critics than citizens—criticizing an effort to improve or change is much easier than leading it or participating in it. For those with fearful or passive-aggressive elements in their personalities, change often elicits latent resistance or hostility.

> People will find 1,000 ingenious ways to withhold cooperation
> from a process that they feel is unnecessary or wrong-headed.
> —John Kotter (2002)

As Kotter's observation suggests, the effective flow leader must understand and become an expert at dealing with resistance and getting at least the key people on board: "There is room for everybody, but the train is leaving the station."

To lead change successfully, you as the leader must be part of the solution. It will not be enough to say, "Here are the new rules." Few of us have the luxury of being able to say, like Captain Jean-Luc Picard of the *Starship Enterprise*, "Make it so!" You will need to establish intrinsic motivation and to involve the key stakeholders. You will need to answer the question, "What's in it for me?" for every participant, from administrators to housekeepers. The staff must buy into the process of change and see how it will make their mission and their work easier. This insight is critical to the effective leader: All meaningful and lasting change is *intrinsically*, not *extrinsically*, motivated. "Do it because I'm the boss!" results in grudging and temporary compliance, if that. "Work with me on this because it makes your job easier—and your patients' lives better" results in deep, fundamental, and lasting change. Thus, boundary management and stakeholder analysis are key skills for the flow leader. (Recommended readings on these skills are listed at the end of this chapter.)

Rewards and Incentives

A number of institutions have found that systems of rewards can help initiate and sustain good flow behaviors. Some are direct and visible rewards; for example, one ED used movie tickets to reward staff for executing new flow behaviors. Beyond the tangible gifts and prizes, however, there are two deeper and often underappreciated and underrated rewards that encourage and support good flow behaviors.

The first is individual feedback through feedback loops, which allow people to identify and emulate effective behaviors and to recognize improvement. Changing behavior can be difficult. As Mark Twain noted, "Nothing so needs reforming as other people's habits." How do you change behaviors that need changing? To change the way doctors and nurses practice, one of the best ways is to compare their performance to that of their peers. This is a powerful motivating tool, a strategy that is often more effective than education, cost reduction, or even the quest for excellence. How does one change physician practice? Show them the data on their performance and compare them to their peers. Physicians want to be at least in the middle or one standard deviation above the norm. (Like all of the schoolchildren in Lake Wobegon, everybody is above average.) Practice evidence-based medicine and then focus on moving the entire bell-shaped curve. Monitor and measure your clinicians' results and present these results through blind or coded anonymous practitioner-specific data. Then concentrate on education and creating tools and processes to make it easy to "do the right thing." Again, focus on moving the entire bell-shaped curve.

The second underappreciated reward is implicit: a job made easier or improved performance that is highly visible. Most healthcare workers are motivated and disciplined and recognize when improved processes translate into improved efficiency and effectiveness in the performance of their roles and tasks. Healthcare workers often enter the field because of a desire to excel and to make a difference in the world. The best and most sustained rewards may be those that enhance the ability of the healthcare worker to make that difference. Intrinsic motivation and rewards are the most sustainable of all.

Ensure Physician Leadership

Physicians are particularly valuable allies in the quest for change. Leaders are not likely to achieve system-level improvement without the enthusiasm, knowledge, cultural clout, and personal leadership of physicians. This commitment requires *alignment of mission and incentives* between the hospital and its physicians. Frequent and clear communication is of supreme importance.

In the initiative that improved flow in the ORs at St. John's Regional Health Center, for example, physician commitment made all the difference. As the vice president of perioperative services, Christina Dempsey (2004), observed, "Very strong physician leadership ... helps determine the vision and goals [of the unit, and] hearing the proposal [to set aside one OR for unscheduled surgeries] from a fellow surgeon was key to their willingness to consider it." Her observations are underscored by those of the system president, Robert Brodhead. "A strong physician advocate is essential when proposing change of this nature," he says. "Don't try this without a strong physician champion" (IHI 2004).

One of the keys to motivating and leading physicians is that they almost universally respond to hard data, particularly if they have had a role at the outset in deciding what data will be monitored. As the adage says, "If they're not with you on the takeoff, they won't be with you on the landing." Get key physician leaders involved early and often. Let them decide what data to monitor and what is appropriate statistical supervision. Identify the key physician thought leader who is most likely to influence attitudes on the change initiative, and involve her on the flow team.

The Flow Team Structure

As the St. John's experience illustrates, administrative commitment to flow initiatives and high-level participation in decision making and follow-through drives successful change. Everybody involved in the change has to be on board. Change to improve flow requires high-quality leadership among both the physician staff and nursing staff, as well as a good team of ED physicians, nurses, and support service personnel. Leadership participation from areas throughout the hospital is critical. The flow team needs to have best-in-class clinical leadership, which is a key driver of performance. A high-quality clinical team that is well trained, ethical, flexible, and fun to be around is also crucial. In the model for a hospital-wide patient flow team structure, high-level administrators join physicians and other clinical leaders on each work team (Figure 4.2). This is an essential feature of the model, and without it the opportunity for success will be limited.

Along with administrative and physician commitment, you will need a local champion for any of the improvement efforts. Initially, work with the innovators, early adapters, and early majority group, identifying allies and change agents (Figure 4.3). When looking for the sources of power and influence, don't ignore the early vocal resisters; once converted, they can be your best champions. According to Collins (2001), Level 5 leaders focus first on the "who," then on the "what." Following this pattern, leaders should first:

- focus on getting the right people on the bus, the wrong people off the bus, and the right people in the right seats;
- *then* figure out where to drive the bus.

Leadership for Patient Flow   85

Figure 4.2. Patient Flow Team Structure

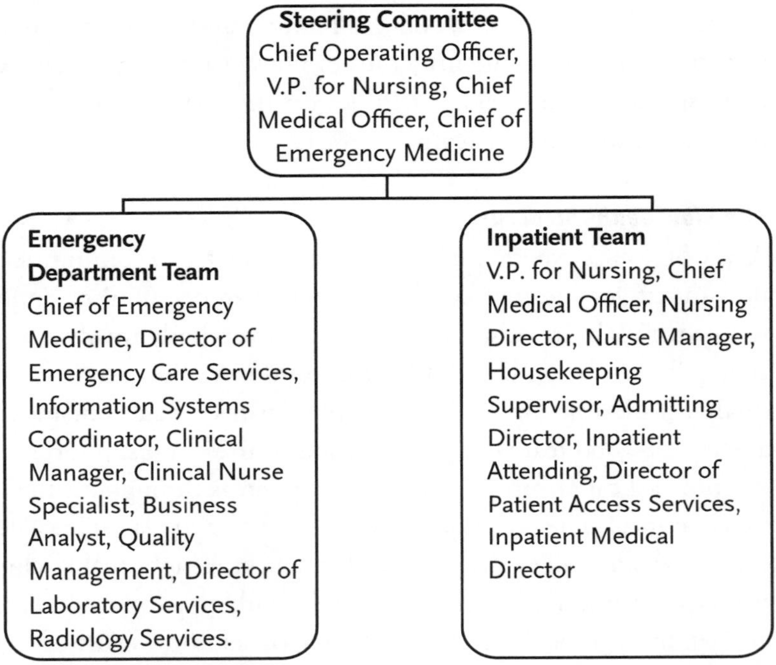

Steering Committee
Chief Operating Officer, V.P. for Nursing, Chief Medical Officer, Chief of Emergency Medicine

Emergency Department Team
Chief of Emergency Medicine, Director of Emergency Care Services, Information Systems Coordinator, Clinical Manager, Clinical Nurse Specialist, Business Analyst, Quality Management, Director of Laboratory Services, Radiology Services.

Inpatient Team
V.P. for Nursing, Chief Medical Officer, Nursing Director, Nurse Manager, Housekeeping Supervisor, Admitting Director, Inpatient Attending, Director of Patient Access Services, Inpatient Medical Director

Source: Adapted from "Bursting at the Seams," Whitepaper from *Urgent Matters* and The George Washington University Medical Center, September 2004. Used with permission.

As you work to lead change, keep the whole process as transparent as possible. Stay on message and realize that there will always be resistance. Sometimes leaders have to transfer the hardcore resisters. You can't please everybody, and some people will be hurt or adversely affected by the change. "Never try to teach a pig to sing. It wastes your time—and it annoys the pig" (North Carolina proverb).

The goal is to organize and bind the team around a common purpose. To accomplish this goal, leaders need to be willing and able to:

- coach and mentor;
- push through key barriers;

Figure 4.3. The Adoption of Change

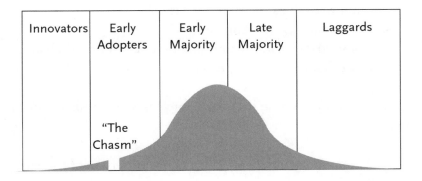

| Innovators | Early Adopters | Early Majority | Late Majority | Laggards |

"The Chasm"

- establish stretch aims or stretch goals;
- stay in touch with the improvement efforts; and
- visit the team and be sure that the team has the resources and support it needs.

In short, leaders need to commit time, resources, and people. As a leader of change, you will meet with a lot of "Nos," so you have to be optimistic and encouraging. Followers want comfort, stability, and solutions to their problems. At times real leaders do need to ask the hard questions and push for results. At times people will be pushed out of their comfort zones, and then you must manage the resulting stress (or distress). Occasionally you will have to circle around and pick up the stragglers, but understand that sometimes you have to leave the unwilling behind.

While it is an essential component of success, enthusiasm alone is not enough to carry an individual department or hospital through the implementation of the necessary changes. Adapting John Kotter's principles for leading change (Kotter 2002), we suggest the following sequence as an order of priority:

1. Establish a sense of urgency.
2. Form a powerful guiding coalition.

3. Create a vision.
4. Communicate the vision.
5. Empower others to act on the vision.
6. Plan for and create short-term wins.
7. Consolidate improvements and produce still more change.
8. Institutionalize new approaches.

At times, situations in healthcare force us to establish a sense of urgency:

- A community experiences the frequent diversion of patients.
- A newly minted patient satisfaction score informs you that patients are unhappy with your services.
- Patients experience unwelcome delays in getting to the operating room or to the catheterization lab.
- A shortage of nurses stresses staff and clinical operations.
- A specialty surgical hospital opens in your area.
- An ED across town closes.

For example, a colleague of the authors' had the following experience. In January, 1997, he was managing the operating room in a large community hospital in North Carolina. Although he had been happily entrenched in his professional silo, our colleague was enticed to join the ED for a "wonderful management opportunity." He walked into this opportunity only to find out that 32 percent of the RN positions were vacant, and the department was without a manager and an assistant manager. The throughput times for the ED were extremely high, and morale was at a low ebb. He then found out after just five days on the job that the only other ED in the area was going to close in two weeks, bringing 14,000 extra patients per year to the department. What to do? You can react in several different ways to an event like this: you can blame, whine, or run, or you can view the situation as an opportunity to make a difference.

Communication is key in leading change. As Kotter's list suggests, there is a compelling need to communicate the vision and to establish urgency, which has a plan, rather than anxiety, which doesn't. Establishing urgency is done in a number of ways across multiple channels. Chief among them is communication, communication, communication.

Effectively Diagnose Problems and Test Changes

With the flow team in place, look at how the system functions and ask the following question: What about the system's processes and practices encourages the results, and what needs to be changed? At St. John's, for example, hourly patient flow analysis revealed—much to everyone's amazement—that the elective surgery stream, not the unscheduled surgeries, was causing the flow problems. When facilitating change, multiple methods or models are useful. We have had particular success with the Rapid Cycle Testing model as initially proposed by Langley, Nolan, and colleagues at Associates for Process Improvement (Langley et al. 1996). It is simple, easy to master, and easy to teach to everyone involved in the change management effort. It involves asking three questions, with three requirements:

Question	Requirement
1) What are we trying to accomplish?	1) A clear statement of change or purpose
2) How will we know that the change is an improvement?	2) Measures
3) What changes can we make that will result in an improvement?	3) A tool kit

A test of change is run, results are noted, modifications are made, and the process starts all over again. The goal is test and learn, test and learn. Changes should be SMART—specific, measurable, actionable, relevant, and time-specific. For example, when St. John's implemented a one-month trial of their OR flow solution, they agreed that if the change didn't improve things, they would return to the old pattern and think of another solution to test. Follow their lead—make the change and see what you discover. If change is an art and resistance is a science, managing change is an art, a science, and a craft.

Change Your Culture and Your Processes

Leading an organization through change not only *can* be hazardous, it almost always *is* hazardous since it involves changing the culture and the way things are done. *Who Moved My Cheese?* (Johnson 1998) is tame compared to this level of change: improving flow in healthcare systems is about changing how and why the work is done. It is about much more than just the money. Changing culture means changing people's lives. People frequently get very unhappy about having their lives changed, even when the change will ultimately benefit them. As comedian Albert Brooks observed: "I don't really mind change. I mind being changed."

The culture you want in your healthcare system that supports changes to improve flow has very specific characteristics:

- a commitment to common goals;
- the espoused values as the system's real values;
- common language and common mental models;
- teamwork, or a sense of looking out for each other and the goals of the team; and
- team member accountability to each other and to the team's goals.

Leaders who want to transform their organizational culture create a dialog for problem solving around the issues of general problem identification, solution formulation, planning, and implementation. Systems thinking is critical to the transformation process, coupled with a set of measures that engage and monitor the entire system. Efforts to improve patient flow need to involve patients, clinical leadership, quality leadership, and hospital leadership. Leaders engage the flow team in identifying the changes that are required and involve the team in preparing for change and planning the change process. To facilitate change, an effective leader must:

- make it easy to say "yes";
- plan for the conditions that are necessary to succeed; and
- build in intrinsic, not just extrinsic, rewards.

Working together with your flow team, implement the changes and then work to sustain them. As your healthcare system undertakes cultural change, expect to address political and personal issues and to deal with competing agendas for time, energy, and resources. Since money, of course, is always an issue, project management is critical. Last, but certainly not least, as you and your team transform your health system's culture into one that serves its patients, staff, and management, celebrate team successes and reward the people who make them possible.

Improved patient flow is necessary for excellence in patient safety and satisfaction, staff satisfaction, and improved financial performance. While the science and methodology will provide the concepts for change-making, the will to execute is fundamental to success. Is leading change challenging? Yes. There are technical (procedural) changes and adaptive (human factors) changes as you cross boundaries and shake up the status quo in culture, structures, and processes. Undertaking this journey, you will face challenges and you will make mistakes. Will the outcome be worth the struggle? You bet!

> How can anyone doubt that a small group of dedicated people can change the world? Indeed, it is the only thing that ever has.
> —Margaret Mead

References

Ackoff, R. 1981. *Creating the Corporate Future*. St. Louis, MO: John Wiley and Sons.

Ambrose, S. 2001. *Band of Brothers: E Company, 506th Regiment, 101st Airborne from Normandy to Hitler's Eagle's Nest*. New York: Simon & Schuster.

Bennis, W. 2003. *On Becoming a Leader*. New York: Perseus Books.

Block, P. 2001. *The Answer to "How" Is "Yes": Acting on What Matters*. San Francisco: Berrett-Koehler.

Collins, J. 2001. *Good to Great*. New York: HarperCollins.

Institute for Healthcare Improvement. 2004. "Improving Surgical Flow at St. John's Regional Health Center: A Leap of Faith." [Online article; retrieved 9/26/06.] http://www.ihi.org/IHI/Topics/Flow/PatientFlow/ImprovementStories/ImprovingSurgicalFlowatStJohnsRegionalHealthCenterSpringfieldMOALeapofFaith.htm

Johnson, S., and K. Blanchard. 1998. *Who Moved My Cheese? An Amazing Way to Deal with Change in Your Work and in Your Life*. New York: Putnam Adult.

Kotter, J. 2002. *The Heart of Change*. Boston: Harvard Business School Press.

Langley, G .L., K. M. Nolan, T. W. Nolan, C. L. Norman, and L. P. Provost. 1996. *The Improvement Guide: A Practical Approach to Enhancing Organizational Performance*. San Francisco: Jossey-Bass Publishers.

Lewin, K. 1948. *Resolving Social Conflicts: Selected Papers on Group Dynamics*. New York: Harper & Row.

Further Recommended Readings

Heifetz R. A., and M. Linsky. 2002. *Leadership on the Line: Staying Alive Through the Dangers of Leading*. Boston: Harvard Business School Press.

Hirschorn, L., and T. Gilmore. 1992. "The New Boundaries of the Boundaryless Company." *Harvard Business Review* 70: 104–115.

Schein, E. H. 1993. "How Can Organizations Learn Faster? The Challenge of Entering the Green Room." *Sloan Management Review* Winter: 85–92.

Winters, R. B. 2006. *Beyond Band of Brothers: The War Memoirs of Major Dick Winters*. New York: Berkeley Press.

CHAPTER 5

The Science of Flow

Make things as simple as possible, but no simpler.

—Albert Einstein

Discovery consists of seeing what everybody has seen and thinking what nobody has thought.

—Albert von Szent-Gyorgyi

IN OUR QUEST to improve flow, as in our quest to lead change effectively, we fortunately don't have to reinvent the wheel. We can build our own strategies on the foundations established by innovators who share our same goals. Creative leaders, as well as business and industry theorists, have developed strategies for streamlining their companies and workplaces, working toward the same efficiency, enjoyment, and service that we seek in our healthcare systems. We can begin by seeing how these theories can be adapted to our own context.

We can also build on the experiences of those in other healthcare systems as we work toward establishing common goals and common measurements for knowing when we have met them. How do we know when the theories we have adopted are resulting in beneficial change? How does what we are doing stack up to what another system has accomplished or what the ideal is for a service? The answer is metrics—measuring our performance.

THEORY—BUT NOT TOO MUCH

Companies such as Disney, the Ritz-Carlton, Nordstrom, Toyota, and Starbucks have built their reputations using the science of flow to deliver almost legendary efficiency and customer service. As pointed out in the business case discussion, healthcare is a personal service business; therefore, a number of the theories and disciplines that these successful service companies use apply equally well to healthcare systems. Some of these techniques—variation and variability, forecasting, demand-capacity management, queuing theory, and the theory of constraints—are particularly relevant to patient flow (Figure 5.1).

Variation and Variability

Variation exists in all of nature and allows for the wonderful differences we see in the environment and in people. This is referred to as natural or random variation. Variation exists in the interests, wants, and even demands of customers and patients. If you ever stood in line at a Starbucks coffee shop, you know it can be difficult just to pronounce a choice, let alone make one from the myriad combinations. In the case of an upscale grocery store, such as Stew Leonard's in Connecticut ("the world's largest dairy store"), not only are the choices seemingly limitless but the customers are unscheduled, and the product is perishable.

In business, random variation is present in the tastes of customers, characteristics of the raw materials, differing skills of employees, and so on. In healthcare, random variation is present in the variety of patient conditions, personalities of individuals, responses to therapy, and rate of the arrival of patients to the ED, operating room, or inpatient unit. This type of variation cannot be eliminated but should be planned for and managed whenever possible. Where differences in clinician skills exist, education and training can create common competencies.

Yet another kind of variation often wreaks havoc with the healthcare system: artificial variation. Artificial or nonrandom variation is often driven by individual priorities that cannot be known or predicted with any regularity. The determination of elective surgical scheduling is an example of artificial variation. Elective surgical schedules are often fully booked on Tuesdays and Thursdays but quite open on Fridays, determined by surgeon preferences rather than actual demand. Another concept that influences the variation of both the total hospital and individual unit census is batching. This is when work (i.e., lab tests and x-ray studies or hospital admissions or discharges) is grouped or batched rather than evenly distributed. Batching has a significant effect on patient flow ("the pig in the python"), but this effect is often disguised by the use of averages as a way to display patient volume or service capacity. Consider the following example:

> Sixteen patients require heart surgery this week. Since the cardiac surgeon prefers to operate on Tuesdays and Thursdays, she schedules eight cases on each day. Patients who have undergone heart surgery must spend at least two days in the ICU postoperatively. Thus, the ICU receives eight patients from cardiac surgery every Tuesday and Thursday.
>
> This clustering of patients usually creates chaos as staff scramble to find space for the surgical patients and those coming to the ICU from the ED, as well as for the patients who currently occupy the beds. If beds cannot be found, then the ED must divert critically ill patients to other facilities. Additional surgical cases requiring postoperative care in the ICU must be cancelled. This peak in volume created by the batch scheduling method affects all areas of the hospital

as patients are shifted in and out of units to make way for the cardiac surgical patients. This is treated as a crisis, yet it happens every week.

Because surgical volume is light near the end of the week, the ICU volume will decrease over the weekend, creating a valley. The seesaw effect of managing these peaks and valleys prevents efficient distribution of the hospital's most limited resources: staff, space, and services. Because elective surgeries are actually scheduled and known in advance, we would expect a relatively smooth demand and little or no census variability. Instead, the variability in hospital census due to elective surgical volume is as great as that created by admissions from the ED.

If the patients requiring cardiac surgery were scheduled over four days, thereby smoothing the surgical flow, the ICU would need to accommodate only four patients each surgical day, allowing for optimal scheduling and predictable demand for staffing and patient beds. The flow of other patients in and out of the ICU is smoother and less stressful for staff and patients. In both cases—batching and smoothing—the surgical volume remains the same, yet the effect on the organization is vastly different.

To find such sources of backup in your own system, map variation in census by time of the day and day of week. Look at the difference between midnight and midday census (or the difference in census between any same-day interval) to determine within-day variation. The difference is often a sign of the mismatch between patient admissions and timely discharges. For between-day variation, the organization can measure the difference between elective surgical admissions or ED admissions expressed either as a standard deviation or as residual differences between days.

Forecasting Future Demand: Guess Who's Coming to Dinner?

In high school, one of the authors worked at a steak house across from a small-town horse arena. In mid-June, the arena owners put up a sign that read: "Horse Show, July 4." We drove by this sign every day. The week before the holiday, the manager gave the day off to all but a skeleton crew, saying, "We're never busy on the Fourth of July." You can guess what happened next: a lot of people waited a really long time for their coffee. The exhausted hostess/waitress/cook's assistant/one-woman bus crew at one point asked incredulously, "Where did all these people come from?" The answer was simple: "From across the street."

You can bet that the staff at Disney World doesn't look out the window on the first day of Easter vacation and say, "Where did all these people come from?" They know they are coming because they came last year and the year before that and the year before that. They have predicted their arrival. Disney may have to factor in gas prices or hurricane threats, but they know about how many people to expect on any given day, and they have contingency plans for variations.

In healthcare, however, we often handle the flow of patients in hospitals or office practices on a minute-to-minute basis, which requires constant triage and crisis management skills. We do this because we believe the actual flow of patients cannot be known and thus planned for in advance. In truth, robust estimates of patient demand, as well as injury types, can be developed using forecasting methodology. In other words, if, like Disney, we look at our data, *we already know who's coming and when.*

Forecasting can use either qualitative (expert opinion) approaches, quantitative (statistical) approaches, or a combination of both to produce an estimate of future demand. Financial managers have been using forecasting methods for years as a way to predict the effect of cost increases, inflation, and reimbursement rates on hospital budgets. Forecasting can also be used effectively to understand patient demand so that staffing, bed availability, and other services can be ready when needed.

Forecasting is based on historical data—for example, patient census by day of the week, time of day, and season of the year. Determining the variables that most affect your census and patient flow is a matter of expert opinion. If you were to wander down to the ED on a Friday night, you would most likely see an extremely busy area full of patients and staff on the run. If you were to remark that the ED seemed awfully full that night, the staff would quickly confirm that it is like this every Friday night! If this is the case, why does the scene seem so chaotic? This same scenario is played out in almost all areas of the hospital, where you will hear staff exclaim, "Tuesdays are always calmer than Thursdays, but Mondays are the worst!" The data usually support the experience the staff report.

How many Friday nights in the ED or Monday mornings in the OR will it take before we decide that things can be better? How many flu seasons will it take before we decide that next year will be different—with contingencies based on forecasting needs (or on forecasting patient demand for care or services)? In short, "Hope is not a plan" (Cooper 2006).

Forecasting Methods

The three types of forecasting methods that are typically used are statistically derived (quantitative) using historical data as inputs. All of these methods benefit from the addition of expert knowledge (qualitative) when experts are asked to review the data and adjust for new surgical techniques, medications, or improvements to care that will significantly affect admissions and patient flow in the future. The three forecasting methods most commonly used are percent adjustment, a moving average, and setting a trendline.

Regardless of the method chosen, the data used must be accurate and readily available. Most organizations find utilization data derived from billing records to be readily available and an excellent source of information. While software packages have been designed exclusively for developing forecasts, these tend to be unnecessarily complex. Commonly used spreadsheet software is fully able to perform the analysis, and it has the additional benefit of previously developed local expertise. Regardless of the source of the actual forecast, remember the needs of the end user of the information: the frontline manager and staff.

Percent Adjustment

Definition: A best guess of what is going to happen in the future based on the percentage increase or decrease of the previous 12 months of performance.

Assumptions/Limitations: That next year will behave like the one that preceded it. This forecast method is highly useful, but may not take into account the variation introduced by seasonal change or other influences. This prediction can be improved by the use of expert opinion; for example, will a new surgical procedure or technology affect this prediction substantially? (Is there a horse show across the street?) This was certainly the case when laparoscopic surgery and cardiac stents exploded onto the medical scene several years ago.

Example: The surgical unit has had 4,000 admissions this year—an increase of 4 percent over the year before. We forecast that during the coming year the surgical unit will have 4,160 admissions, a 4 percent increase over this year.

Moving Average

Definition: As the title implies, the moving average method averages the number of patient visits for the previous time period. For example, a 12-month moving average patient admission forecast would usethe data from the previous 12 months to forecast the patient admissions for the next month. This method is continued for each new month based on the previous 12-month average.

Assumptions/Limitations: As with the percent adjustment method, no correction may exist for seasonal differences, and the prediction can be improved by the use of expert opinion. The method doesn't take flu season into account, for example. Because it is derived as an average, it is not sensitive to monthly shifts, whether up or down.

Example: If you were to forecast the number of patients to be admitted to the ICU in January 2007, you would use the average number of ICU admissions from the previous 12 months (December 2005 to December 2006).

Trendline

Definition: A best-fit line that is statistically derived using regression analysis based on historical data. It answers the question: "How good was our planning against the actual number of admissions in the previous 12 months?" The "goodness of fit" of one line against the other allows you to make stronger predictions going forward.

Assumptions/Limitations: This is a more accurate method than the first two but still assumes that recent trends will continue. It will take a little more explaining than either the percent adjustment or the 12-month moving average. As with the two previous examples, the trendline can be derived using any commonly available spreadsheet program. Your financial analysts will be very familiar with this tool—ask them for help!

Example: If you were to forecast the number of patients to be admitted to the ICU in January 2007, you would use the information from the trendline analysis to check for accuracy of prediction or to correct current predictions up or down.

Note: There is a special case of the trendline that adjusts for seasonality. It is more complex but more accurate, especially if your healthcare system experiences large and predictable shifts in flow throughout the year.

The fact that unscheduled demand can actually be modeled (or described) and forecasted is an unbelievably advantageous tool for the healthcare industry. However, this tool is glaringly underused, if used at all.

Demand-Capacity Management

Once we have an idea what the demand will be, how do we match capacity to it? Service capacity is a perishable commodity. Unlike products stored in warehouses for future consumption, a service is an intangible personal experience that cannot be transferred from one person to another. Instead, a service is produced and consumed at the same time. Whenever the demand for a health-care service falls short of the capacity to serve, the results are doctors playing video games and OR rooms standing empty. On the other hand, when demand exceeds capacity, we have stacked-up patients, overburdened providers, and too little space. Further, the variability in service demand, especially in healthcare, can be quite pronounced. The problem can be approached from two different directions: smoothing consumer demand or matching service capacity to meet the demand. Both strategies are data driven and are only recently being explored in the medical arena.

Demand requires a bit of smoothing because of human behavior. We like to take our meals at roughly the same time of day and our vacations in the summer months. We often show up at restaurants at 7:30 p.m., for example, and often head for the seaside hotels in July. This makes for idle periods and consumer waiting. In the ED, the system is stressed most during the evening hours, on Saturdays and Mondays, and on holidays. Some EDs may vary in volume by almost 50 percent from one day to the next. Because they confront the same kinds of peaks and valleys, service industries have developed strategies to help match capacity to demand—strategies equally useful in healthcare settings. Scheduling can help smooth demand, while customer participation, cross training, and sharing capacity can help meet that demand (Figure 5.2).

Scheduling

One business strategy that can help smooth demand is the promotion of off-peak service. We're all familiar with this approach. You can get a really cheap trip to the Bahamas in the summer, and you can save money with the "early bird special" in some restaurants if you eat dinner before 5 p.m. Your phone company likely reduces its rates for late-night calling. This strategy can be adapted to medical service as well. For example, some EDs that see patients in follow-up for dressing changes or further tests will

Figure 5.2. Demand Capacity Management Stratigies

1. Scheduling
2. Customer participation
3. Cross training
4. Shared capacity

---

try to steer these patients to the low-volume hours and attract them with the promise of faster throughput. A healthcare system, for example, might consider reduced copays for early morning ED visits. Another ED that brings patients back for the tests that are unavailable in the ED at night has negotiated the first ultrasound appointment in the morning and the first stress-test appointment for ED patients. This "scheduling" in off hours again helps smooth demand. This concept can be applied in a similar fashion to elective surgery or to the demand for outpatient services.

Even when demand is smoothed, we will still need other strategies for matching capacity to demand. Building *flexibility* into the system is a key to managing peak loads and to being prepared for the unexpected spikes in demand that will occur despite good forecasting. Sharing the responsibility for tasks helps keep work from piling up and helps ensure smooth flow.

Customer Participation

Pump-your-own gas, the self-serve grocery checkout, and the fix-your-own coffee bar all encourage people to do for themselves something an employee used to do for them. While we aren't suggesting start-your-own IVs or take-your-own x-rays, patients and families can take on some of the routine tasks that healthcare staff used to do for them. For example, family members can participate in patient care. We see this model in systems like the Mayo Clinic, where hotel-like facilities substitute for hospital beds. Patients can be given materials to set up their own follow-up appointments, thus freeing staff from these administrative tasks. An emerging trend in the ED is the "diagnostic waiting room," where family members work with ED staff to meet the needs of patients waiting to be treated. Customer participation, to which people have become more and more accustomed, is another tool in the demand-capacity management toolbox, and having families and patients take more responsibility for their care across the healthcare continuum is a trend that is likely to continue.

Cross Training

Another task-sharing demand capacity strategy adapted from successful business is cross training. Having employees who know how to work in more than one area can be liberating for both the system and the staff. For example, the night before Mother's Day at the local upscale grocery store, the store manager was happily (it seemed, anyway) making floral arrangements alongside his floral manager, who was overwhelmed with requests. The store manager's skill level indicated that this was not his first time, as he was quite accomplished. He gave the impression that he could just as easily have been weighing fish, if he needed to be.

While the skills required for hospital cross training are certainly more complex, the same principle applies. Staff members are trained in multiple skills to meet the fluctuations in demand. For example, nurses are trained to do respiratory therapy or ED technicians are trained to start IVs. A related strategy is specialty training for staff members. For example, nurses can be trained and certified as laceration specialists or forensic nurse examiners in the ED. Extending the skills of the staff creates elasticity in the system that is needed when demand is high.

Shared Capacity

A second form of sharing that helps capacity meet demand is sharing space or services. This strategy is particularly adaptable to any area of the hospital that experiences large fluctuations in volume. Nighttime use of adjacent clinic space vacated by 9-to-5 service operations such as day surgery helps some EDs meet their evening peak space demands. Use of the PACU for nighttime ICU overflow has been tried in multiple hospitals. Hallway boarding in the inpatient units is a second form of space sharing that helps use the capacity of the entire system rather than one area of it to relieve pressure and enable provision of better care. We are not so much recommending the use of any of these measures as we are illustrating the importance of the principle. Understanding the principles and applying them to your healthcare system will offer you the most likely avenue for success.

Queuing Theory

No matter how hard we try to manage variability, forecast needs, and match capacity to demand, we will still sometimes have sluggish flow in our healthcare systems. In other words, patients will have to wait for services—wait for tests, wait to be seen by the physician, wait for discharge. A queue will exist. As we explored a bit in the first chapter, Disney is the undisputed master of managing the queue, simply defined for our purposes as a line of people waiting for something: a movie ticket, the dry cleaning, a turn at the copier, an x-ray. We already know one basic queuing rule: when we are in a hurry, we're behind the customer with the coupons and a cart overloaded with groceries. We also know, as explored in Chapter 2, that queuing profoundly affects patient satisfaction and the quality of service we are able to provide. So what can we learn from the service expertise of others?

First, let's take a look at a few principles and terms. Systems serving uncontrolled or unscheduled arrivals behave in a characteristic fashion. When (patient) inflow and service times are random, the healthcare unit's or the healthcare system's response to increasing utilization is nonlinear. As utilization rises above 80 to 85 percent, waits and delays increase exponentially (Figure 5.3). Thus, we can anticipate, for instance, that as hospital occupancy goes up, delays in the ED or the PACU for admissions will increase. Likewise, as the OR schedule approaches capacity, the ability to handle emergency surgery cases is impaired and the ED feels the delays.

Where do the people come from and how do they arrive? The term for the area from which a system draws its customers is its

Figure 5.3. Relationship Between Utilization and Delays

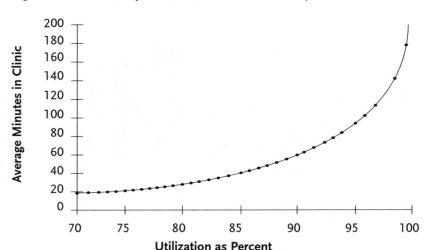

Source: Noon, C. E., C. T. Hankins, and M. J. Cote. 2003. "Understanding the Impact of Variation in the Delivery of Healthcare Services." *Journal of Healthcare Management* 48 (2): 82–98. Used with permission.

calling population, the source of service customers from a market area. The size and makeup of this population are affected by factors such as health insurance, hospital services (such as trauma), and ambulance patterns.

The manner in which this group arrives can be explored through a Poisson distribution, the name for a complex mathematical formula that actually describes or models unscheduled demand for services. It can describe the arrival rate of ED patients by unit of time such as hour of day or day of week (Figure 5.4). This information can help a health-care system predict arrivals in the ED or any unit or entry point that deals with unscheduled patient arrivals or demand for services.

A few other terms are important in describing people's responses to being in the queue for services. A balk is an arriving customer who sees a long line and decides not to seek that service. It is what you do when you see the line out the door at Starbucks and say, "No way am I standing in that," and go to the

Figure 5.4. A Census Distribution

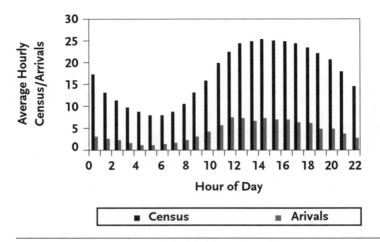

7-Eleven. The ED analog is the LWBS patient. *Reneging* occurs when a customer in a queue departs before obtaining service. The equivalent is the patient who decides to have surgery or a cardiac catheterization elsewhere because scheduling is delayed or cumbersome. If you actually stood in the coffee line for a few minutes before you decided to leave, you are reneging. (Renegers have a touch of optimism.) The ED permutations of reneging are the people who check in, sit a while, look around and see that nobody has moved, and leave, as well as the LBTCs, who may in fact have begun the treatment process before they decide they can't do the wait.

One other pertinent term is queue *discipline*, which is often closely related to reneging. Queue discipline is a rule for selecting the next customer in line to be served. For example, queue discipline is disregarded when the gentleman behind the deli counter ignores you while he takes the orders of three parties of six who came in after you did. Because queue discipline in healthcare is overridden by triage principles, the order in which arrivals are seen is often misunderstood and can be the source of patient complaints where it appears that anything other than a first come, first served model is in place. Hence the connection of queue discipline to reneging: patients may leave before obtaining service if they are dissatisfied with the seeming inequity in the process.

Another important service industry queuing principle for application to healthcare is minimizing and managing the waits. Disney excels at making the wait feel as short as possible and making the customer feel that the wait was not so bad, which involves both managing expectations and providing diversions. Healthcare can do the same. First, minimize the wait by using demand-capacity management tools to predict who is coming and when and to have resources at the ready: we are fully staffed, our Fast Track is open and our operating rooms are ready, and we have a plan for overflow (Full Capacity Protocol, a backup surgical team and OR, for example). When patients must wait, help manage the time: we provide a pleasant environment and instructional and entertaining materials to help patients feel more relaxed, and we manage expectations by keeping patients informed as they wait (see Chapter 2, "How Patients Win"). A concierge in the ED, the provision of beepers for patients and families, and the installation of computer jacks, for example, can all improve the wait for our patients in queue.

Furthermore, because we know—or could choose to know—when our patients will be arriving, we have the capacity and the ability (but often not the will) to predict queuing delays. Hospitals that employ a "Green Light—Go!; Yellow Light—Slow!; Red Light—No (at least not now)!" system (see Chapter 6 for more information) understand this concept and put it in use for their staff—and their patients. Patient flow is a network of queues and bottlenecks (both relative and absolute), which leads us to the theory of constraints.

Theory of Constraints

The theory of constraints is a management philosophy that focuses on finding the scarce resources or weakest links in a service chain, and identifying it as the constraint on the system. In the flower-shipping business, for example, mainline refrigerated trucks follow a north-south pattern, running from Miami to New York. To truck flowers north from eastern North Carolina, they have to be transported to Miami, a constraint on a smaller operation's system. Healthcare has its own constraints, with each system having its own weaknesses. Perhaps the constraint is not enough nurses or turnaround times that are too long. To use the theory of constraints to improve flow, go through four focusing steps:

1. Identify the system's constraint(s):
   - What limits productivity of the entire system?
   - Look for a long queue of work or long processing times.
2. Decide how to exploit the system's constraints:
   - Make decisions on how to modify or redesign the task/activity/process so that work may be performed more effectively.
3. Subordinate everything else to the decisions made in step 2:
   - Make implementing step 2 one of your highest priorities.
4. Elevate the system's constraints:
   - Add capacity (more physicians, more nurses, more beds?) or off-load demand (can someone or something else do this or can it be done elsewhere?).

If in the previous step a constraint has been broken, go back to step 1, but do not allow inertia to cause a new constraint. Set up a process of ongoing improvement. A new bottleneck will always be identified. Follow the above steps to improve or eliminate this new bottleneck. Remember, an hour lost at a *bottleneck* in the process is an hour lost for the entire system. Time saved at a *non-bottleneck* is a mirage.

A real constraint—a physician, a nurse, a hospital bed, an OR—is a valuable resource that should be used to the fullest. Constraints should neither be exhausted nor idle. Any constraint should be doing work that only constraints should do. Physicians should not be parking cars or opening the mail, for instance. Less obviously, you don't want nurses being administrative assistants. Look at the actual tasks that a key member of the team who is a scarce resource performs to determine which tasks are best done by her and which should be off-loaded or, better yet, eliminated.

Constraints or bottlenecks in healthcare systems can be addressed in the following ways:

- Identify: Find the longest processing times. In the emergency department, for example, are people waiting too long?
- Exploit: Redesign the system for more efficiency. For example, add a Fast Track to handle nonacute patients, implement Adopt-a-Boarder to free up needed beds, use team triage to accelerate the decision-making process, and so on.
- Subordinate: Make a matrix of the processes with the longest times and work to eliminate the delays one by one. If radiology turnaround times delay patients, assign a designated x-ray technician for the ED and/or empower nurses and midlevel providers to order x-rays at first contact with the patient.
- Elevate: Use midlevel providers, such as scribes, and template charting to off-load paperwork and to free nurses to work with patients.

Keep teams working to optimize flow by looking out for new or relative bottlenecks and begin the process all over again.

Rapid Cycle Improvement

Improvement can be accelerated by intense focus on a specific subject and by maintaining support for rapidly conducted, small-scale "tests of change" in plan-do-study-act (PDSA) cycles. Three specific ideas are at the heart of rapid cycle improvement: the Model for Improvement; the PDSA cycle; and change concepts.

The Model for Improvement

The Model for Improvement was first presented by Langley and colleagues (1992) in *The Foundation of Improvement*, where they observed that organizations able to make rapid gains seem to have an underlying capacity to answer three questions, and to set in place small-scale tests of change guided by their answers to those questions:

1. What are we trying to accomplish?
2. How will we know if a change is an improvement (especially from the viewpoint of the customer)?
3. What changes that we make will result in an improvement?

The Plan-Do-Study-Act Cycle

The ability to run tests of change is intimately associated with sound improvement. This ability is codified in the language of quality improvement as the PDSA cycle (Figure 5.5). PDSA cycles are key to the improvement process and must be strongly emphasized. The pace of testing is crucial—running small cycles soon is better than running large ones after a long time. Each cycle, properly done, is informative and provides a basis for further improvement. In some important sense, the more cycles, the more learning.

Depending on their aim, teams choose promising changes and use PDSA cycles to test a change quickly on a small scale, see how it works, and refine the change as necessary before implementing it on a broader scale. The following example shows how a team started with a small-scale test.

- **Plan:** Ask one nurse to see if he can, in consultation with the patient, assign a scheduled time for the patient to go home, and meet that time within 30 minutes.

Figure 5.5. PDSA Cycle

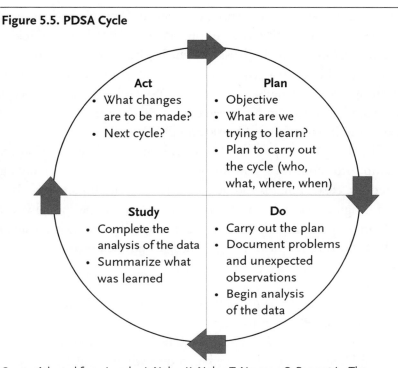

Act
- What changes are to be made?
- Next cycle?

Plan
- Objective
- What are we trying to learn?
- Plan to carry out the cycle (who, what, where, when)

Study
- Complete the analysis of the data
- Summarize what was learned

Do
- Carry out the plan
- Document problems and unexpected observations
- Begin analysis of the data

Source: Adapted from Langley J, Nolan K, Nolan T, Norman C, Provost L., The Improvement Guide. (San Francisco: Jossey-Bass 1996), p.60. Used with permission.

- **Do:** The nurse and patient agree on 1:30 p.m. as the scheduled time for the patient to go home, and the patient is discharged at 1:40 p.m.
- **Study:** The patient was happy to be included in the decision, the family was thrilled that they could plan in advance when to be there to pick up the patient, the care team all knew the schedule and were able to work toward the goal, and the nurse found the goal helped organize the work.
- **Act:** The nurse will test this change with three patients tomorrow.

Change Concepts

All improvements involve changes; but not all change is improvement. The changes tested in PDSA cycles should be "smart changes," informed by theory, logic, or prior experience. These change concepts are general ideas—with proven or predicted merit and a sound scientific foundation—on the basis of which ideas for specific process changes can be constructed. As a theoretically grounded idea used to organize a series of tangible small-scale PDSA cycles, a change concept is the driving connection between each small change an organization makes and its larger goal of breakthrough improvement.

The change concept is the theoretically grounded idea for change. Examples for improving flow include, do tasks in parallel, use forcing functions, create pull instead of push systems, and display data visually for tighter control. The "process change" is the specific, physical realization of the idea that is subjected to specific testing on a small scale. Following are three change concepts and the process change to test.

1. *Do tasks in parallel.* Test: Clean the OR while the team is prepping the next patient.
2. *Create a pull system.* Test: Schedule discharges and call the ED, letting them know when rooms will be available throughout the day.
3. *Use forcing functions.* Test: Make it impossible to connect a feeding tube to an IV line.

The theories considered in this chapter are not new, but their application in the clinical setting relative to patient flow is innovative. Many success stories can be found in service industries, and healthcare practitioners and managers need to leverage that knowledge and apply those tools. On a recent business trip, I arrived at my hotel frazzled, tired, and stressed. My plane was late; my taxi took too long—then got lost. When I reached the front desk a cheerful check-in clerk said, "Good evening, Dr. Jensen—we've been expecting you!" Did it change my night? Absolutely! Should it happen at your hospital? You bet it should!

If you want to have some fun, carefully learn and understand the principles, ideas, and models described in this chapter and elsewhere and then visit other service industries to see what you observe that can be applied in your institution. Another variation of this practice is to pay attention to these principles every time you interact with another service industry (restaurants, telephone call centers, dry cleaners, retail outlets, gas stations) and see what you observe that can reinforce what you are doing well in your institution or identify opportunities and techniques for improvement.

Is the day coming when patients make "scheduled appointments" for a limited number of nonacute slots in the ED? Is the day here when admissions and discharges should be slotted into preset times based on historical demand? Will we, like restaurants, take "fax orders" that require a completed demographic and insurance form faxed to the ED to "preregister"? Will somebody say to the patients as they walk through the door, "Welcome—we've been expecting you?" The authors think so. We hope so. Hundreds, perhaps thousands of ideas can be applied from service industries to healthcare today to make this happen—if only we have the will and the daring!

MEASUREMENTS OF SUCCESS

Intuition becomes increasingly valuable in the new information society precisely because there is so much data.

—John Naisbitt

Why is it that we are choking on data, but starved for wisdom?

—Tom Peters

However beautiful the strategy, you should occasionally look at the results.

—Winston Churchill

With our theories in action, how do we know when we are making measurable progress and how do we compare to other healthcare systems that are on the same flow improvement journey? Today, metrics for measuring patient flow performance are often poorly defined and far from standardized. The Institute for Healthcare Improvement has bed turns data available on its website. Several healthcare service organizations (Veteran's Health Administration [VHA], Premier, the Advisory Board, the Medical Group Management Association [MGMA]), specialty societies, and select consulting firms have benchmarking data available for their members or clients. Despite data-accrual efforts by large benchmarking organizations such as the Emergency Department Benchmarking Alliance (EDBA), the VHA, and The Robert Wood Johnson Foundation Urgent Matters Project, even the simplest flow benchmarking measures have poorly standardized definitions. Yet these metrics are cited in the literature as markers for quality, efficiency, and good care.

Widespread confusion still exists about data that measure performance and data that define the characteristics of an institution. Some data may reflect performance along certain parameters, but other data are useful when seeking to understand the nature of the practice at that institution and to find appropriate benchmarking partners. This chapter explores a set of measures that will be useful in measuring flow progress. In quest of greater clarity in this area, much recent work has been done on benchmarking principles and standards in emergency medicine, and these will be discussed in some detail here. The principles can be applied to patient flow in any microsystem—the OR, the PACU, the ICU, telemetry, and so on. The current best metrics for global hospital throughput are patient LOS (which can be adjusted for caseload mix and severity) and IHI's bed turns definition and comparisons (IHI 2006). Hospital LOS can also be looked at by a diagnosis-related group (DRG) to get an idea of the flow of various patient segments or patient streams.

Figure 5.6 lists characteristics that may help to stratify hospital EDs for the purpose of finding the appropriate cohort group. At least until a widely accepted cohort scheme is developed, hospitals (even within a single healthcare system) should seek to benchmark

Figure 5.6. Characteristics for Stratification for Emergency Department Benchmarking

- Annual census
- Pediatric volume
- Trauma center designation
- Admission rate
- Urban/suburban/rural location
- Charity care
- Care levels 1 and 2
- Care levels 3–5
- University/teaching status

against facilities with similar characteristics. Small rural hospitals, for example, should benchmark with others that have the same population and profile.

Finding a Benchmarking Partner

Addressing the need for standardized benchmarking guidelines, in February 2006 a group of experts interested in ED benchmarking met in Atlanta and developed a set of definitions and terms, as well as a cohort scheme (EDBA 2006) (Figure 5.7). This meeting generated a consensus document on operational definitions, metrics, and benchmarking. It uses both patient population and care-level capacity to group hospitals for comparative purposes. Using the scheme, EDs should first identify other EDs in hospitals in the same geographic area for benchmarking purposes. Benchmark cohorts would likely be built first at the state level, then at the regional level. For a complete dictionary of benchmarking terms and definitions as set forth by the Atlanta Summit, see Appendix 1.

Overall Performance Measures versus Operational Benchmarks

In addition to the variations in benchmark standards addressed by the summit are differences between overall performance measures and

Figure 5.7. The Atlanta Summit Emergency Department Cohort Scheme

Volume and Acuity	<10,000	10,000– 29,999	30,000– 49,999	>50,000
Low	Trauma – Admission Rate < 20% Transplant –	Trauma – Admission Rate < 20% Transplant –	Trauma 3 or – Admission Rate < 20% Transplant –	Trauma 3 or – Admission Rate < 20% Transplant –
High	Trauma 1,2,3 Admission Rate < 20% Transplant –	Trauma 1,2,3 Admission Rate < 20% Transplant –	Trauma 1,2 Admission Rate < 20% Transplant –	Trauma 1 Admission Rate < 20% Transplant –

Using the Atlanta Summit Cohort Scheme: the annual volume of the ED is used to assign it to one of four volume categories; and the acuity function is applied to designate high or low acuity. These acuity markers and their functions are described in the chart.

operational benchmarks. In the past, measures of performance were often limited to overall TAT (throughput) and AMA rates. Information technology can now analyze data that are more detailed, with performance and operational benchmarks more clearly distinguished. General performance measures include such areas as admission and discharge throughput, walk-away rates, and patient complaint numbers. Operational measures include specific data on subprocesses within these larger components of flow, specifically times from door to doctor, from lab test to result, and from admission to bed placement, for example. Figure 5.8 lists these general performance and operational measures.

Leadership for Smooth Patient Flow

Figure 5.8. Emergency Department Performance and Operational Metrics

Overall Performance Metrics

- Throughput admitted patients
- Throughput discharged patients

- Walk-aways: AMA, LWBS, LBTC, LWOT
- Complaint ratios

Process/Operational Metrics

- Registration throughput
- Triage time
- Door to doctor
- Decision to bed placement

- Radiology turnaround time
- Laboratory turnaround time
- Admission time
- Discharge time

ED throughput may be delayed by any of these operations or processes, and increasingly data are being gathered to identify backlogs, delays, and inefficiencies. Other schemes for breaking down ED flow processes are listed in Figure 5.9.

Information technology is aiding these efforts by assisting with data accrual, with data becoming increasingly specific and accessible. For instance, the VHA has gathered operational data for most ED processes and has drilled down to segment those further: radiology throughput has been broken down to time from doctor to order, order to x-ray, x-ray to reading, and so on (www.vha.com). This type of granularity can assist frontline practitioners who are using the theory of constraints to identify and address steps in the process where bottlenecks occur. For institutions or units that do not have access to this level of detail, data sampling is a powerful tool that can approximate these results. The subject is well described in many basic statistics textbooks, as well as on IHI's web site (www.ihi.org).

Overall Performance Metrics
Throughput (Admitted Patients, Discharged Patients)

Although throughput may also be referred to as LOS, for the ED the preferred term is *throughput* or *TAT*, as LOS connotes days and

Figure 5.9. ED Flow Process Schemes

ABCD	Healthcare Advisory Board	Best Practices
Arrival → Bed	Door to Doctor	Door to Deck
Bed → Clinician	Doctor to Diagnostics	Deck to Doctor
Clinician → Disposition/ Discharge	Diagnostics to Disposition	Doctor to Diagnostics
		Diagnostics to Decision
		Decision to Disposition
		Discharge

Source: Adapted in part from Twanmoh, J. R., and G. P. Cunningham. 2006. "When Overcrowding Paralyzes an Emergency Department." [Online whitepaper; retrieved 9/27/06] http://www.managedcaremag.com

usually refers only to inpatient stays. For the ED, the reference is hours to minutes. The TAT varies with the nature of the hospital. Higher-volume EDs and tertiary care centers have longer TATs, while smaller, lower-acuity EDs may have shorter times. In general, as the admission rate goes up, so does the throughput time, suggesting that admitted patients slow down the ED system. Facilities with significant numbers of boarders can attest to this fact. Although ultimately different benchmarks for different types of EDs will exist, reference points include the following median TATs:

- 1 hour or less for Fast Track discharged patients;
- 2 hours for non–Fast Track discharged patients; and
- 3 hours for admitted patients.

Simply looking at overall TAT, without segmenting for acuity, is an inadequate means to measure flow. Similarly, hospitals that understand flow will also segment their inpatient length of stay by unit, diagnostic group, and acuity, at a minimum.

Number of Walk-aways

Walk-aways may be the least consistently measured metric of the overall measures for flow. In part this inconsistency results from the difficulty of accurately measuring each subset within this metric and in the contamination of data. The distinctions among patients who LWBS, LBTC, LWOT, and AMA are often subtle and difficult to distinguish. Having a single category of patients called "walk-aways" might eliminate some confusion and improve comparative data. This category would include any patient recognized as an ED encounter who leaves before being admitted or discharged formally by the physician. Since all patients in this larger category are high risk from the standpoint of the ED, perhaps one category may be worth considering.

Complaint Ratios

Complaints in the ED generally range from 0.5 to 3 per 1,000 ED visits. Teaching and tertiary care hospitals generally have higher levels of complaints, as do higher-volume EDs. The methodology of collecting and analyzing complaints data is institutionally specific, and the most important thing is to have a consistent complaint management process in place. The analytical process should distinguish the nature of complaints: clinical care, facilities, wait time, and service, for example. To improve flow, you need to know what makes patients dissatisfied in order to address these issues.

Process and Operational Metrics Door to Doctor Time

The door-to-doctor performance measure may be the most critical in terms of ED patient satisfaction and throughput and may have interesting implications for other areas or units of the hospital as well. The faster the patient sees the physician, the less likely it is that the patient will leave before his or her treatment is complete. Delays are better tolerated at the back end of the visit, and patient satisfaction goes up as the door-to-doctor time decreases. Most institutions define the door-to-doctor time as the interval between the point when a patient is recognized as an ED encounter and the point when the patient is seen by the physician. This metric is very useful, but it needs to be studied carefully. For example, if the door-to-doctor time increases significantly, one might easily assume that the solution is more doctors. However, when this metric is segmented by process, a different conclusion may be reached. As Figure 5.10 shows, different methods of data collection

Figure 5.10. Analyzing Door-to-Doctor: Two Scenarios

ED #1

Door to doctor	1 hour(Up from 35 minutes)
Deck to doctor	48 minutes
Problem?	12 minutes
Solution?	Another doctor in ED
Result?	Door to doctor at 40 minutes

ED #2

Door to doctor	1 hour(Up from 35 minutes)
Deck to doctor	48 minutes
Problem?	12 minutes
Solution?	More beds, more RN's on shifts
Result?	Door to doctor at 40 minutes

may lead to different solutions—more doctors in one case, more rooms and nurses in another.

Tracking systems often allow these times to be tracked with little difficulty. A high-performance ED should adjust its processes to facilitate early face-to-face encounters between patients and physicians. The accepted benchmark is under 30 minutes.

Other ED Operations

Neither the exact definitions nor the numerical benchmarks behind other ED operations have been established yet. Definitions and benchmarks will be forthcoming as more and more institutions take on service operations management and adopt a commitment to metric-based management. Numbers don't tell the whole story, but they are a necessary part of improvement. Following are a few take-home points about operational benchmarks:

1. *Registration throughput:* Bedside registration is often superior to traditional registration modes in terms of operational efficiency. Most institutions have realized a 20- to 30-minute

improvement in throughput times with the introduction of bedside registration.

2. *Triage time:* Traditional triage is currently being questioned because of its bottlenecking potential and the view of many thought leaders that it places a barrier between the physician and the patient. Team triage, a doctor in triage, abbreviated triage, and triage to the diagnostic waiting room are all relatively new ideas being evaluated to replace or augment traditional triage and to improve triage times.

3. *Lab TAT:* Several benchmarking groups have proposed 30 minutes as a TAT for a complete blood count, and other specific benchmarks are being sought. A pneumatic tube system, point-of-care testing, an ED lab, a dedicated ED phlebotomist, and bar-coded specimens are all innovations that improve the lab TAT. Contingency plans for backlogs and delays are critical.

4. *Radiology TAT:* Several benchmarking groups have suggested 30–60 minutes as the benchmark for a plain radiograph TAT. Dedicated x-ray technicians, tele-radiography, and voice recognition software have all been associated with improved radiology throughput. Again, contingency plans for backlogs and delays are critical.

5. *Discharge time:* It has been suggested that the discharge process should take under 30 minutes. Preprinted discharge instructions, "To Go" packs, discharge teams, discharge kiosks, and contingency plans all help expedite this process.

6. *Decision to admit to bed placement:* With 75 percent of hospital EDs spending part of every day at overcapacity and admitted patients being boarded in hallways in the ED, the time from decision (to admit) to transporting a patient to an inpatient bed can often be more than 12 hours. Ideally, the goal of less than 2 hours from decision to admit to admission has been suggested. This may vary with the type of hospital, the admission rate, and the acuity of care.

Designating one person with centralized bed authority (a bed "czar" or "czarina") who is responsible for all admissions and transfers, using electronic bed management systems, planning and scheduling discharges, and centralizing housekeeping and transport services can all positively affect this metric.

A WORD ABOUT TECHNOLOGY

As benchmarks for service processes and times are established in healthcare, we will increasingly depend on technology to gather data. Automated systems can track and trend data to show where bottlenecks occur and to measure success in reducing them. Ideally, a real-time dashboard helps track current throughput times for patients and turnaround times for services such as lab and radiology to reduce waste and variability in a timely way (Figure 5.11; see also Chapter 6). A patient flow dashboard can help your healthcare system monitor patient flow on a real-time basis and then implement backup protocols and procedures in real time to alleviate bottlenecks or overburdened units. Patient flow dashboards have proved particularly useful in the ED setting and in managing hospital-wide admissions and transfers, as well as patient flow in specific areas or units. This information allows a sustained focus on service, satisfaction, and quality.

The development of dashboards is a tremendously exciting area, and remarkable improvements are expected in the functionality and usefulness of this technology over the next several years.

Technology should always be marshaled in the service of a simple but important goal—quality, safety, and service. In the ED, key goals include:

- getting the doctor and the patient in a room together as quickly as possible; and

Figure 5.11. Dashboard Technology

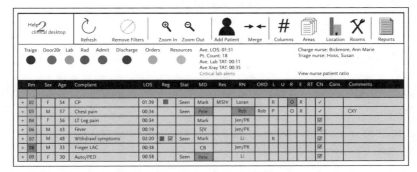

Source: Patient Flow Enewsletter. Volume 2, Issue 6. Thursday, December 8, 2005. Used with permission.

- organizing a service line so that doctors can be doctors and nurses can be nurses (rather than data processors and administrative assistants).

Further, the most sophisticated of these tracking systems save the data in a data mart for mining at a later date. These data sets are being used to better define the elements of flow by numerically mapping out the service cycles of the healthcare system. EDs, for example, are able to track how many patients they see, how long it takes to see them, what resources are used, and whether the patients are admitted. In the not too distant future all healthcare systems should have this type of data available for forecasting and demand capacity management.

A word of caution is wise, however, in considering information technology as a source of success measurement and a solution to flow problems. As James Adams (2006), chair of emergency medicine at Northwestern University in Illinois, succinctly put it, "Information technology can be a false god."

While information technology provides increased accessibility to data, that data must be interpreted and analyzed in a meaningful way to come to sound, systems-focused decisions. "Don't confuse data with knowledge or knowledge with wisdom. All three are important, but the first two must always lead to the third—otherwise they are wasted" (Thom Mayer, M.D.).

References

Adams, J. 2006. Personal communication with Thom Mayer and Kirk Jensen. February.

Cooper, A. 2006. *Dispatches From the Edge: A Memoir of War, Disasters, and Survival.* New York: Harper Collins

Emergency Department Benchmarking Alliance. 2006. Meeting at the Emergency Department Performance Measurement Summit in Atlanta, GA. February 23.

Institute for Healthcare Improvement. 2005. "The Hospital Flow Diagnostic" [Online whitepaper; retrieved 8/24/06.] www.ihi.org/IHI/Topics/Flow/PatientFlow/EmergingContent/HospitalFlowDiagnostic.htm.

Langley, G. J., K. M. Nolan, and T. W. Nolan. 1992. *The Foundation of Improvement.* Silver Spring, MD: API Publishing.

Peters, T. 2006. *Reimagine!: Business Excellence in a Disruptive Age.* London: DK Adult.

Further Recommended Readings

Advisory Board. 2000. "Building the Clockwork ED: Best Practices for Eliminating Bottlenecks and Delays in the ED." Washington, DC : Advisory Board/HWorks.

Fitzsimmons, J., and M. Fitzsimmons. 2006. *Service Management: Operations, Strategy, Information Technology*, 5th ed. Boston: McGraw-Hill.

Goldratt, E. 1986. *The Goal.* Great Barrington, MA: North River Press.

Graff, L., C. Stevens, D. Spaite, and J. Foody. 2002. "Measuring and Improving Quality in Emergency Medicine." *Society for Academic Emergency Medicine* 9 (11): 1091–07.

Holland, L., L. Smith, and K. Blick. 2005. "Reducing Laboratory Turnaround Time Outliers Can Reduce Emergency Department Patient Length of Stay." *American Journal of Clinical Pathology* 125 (5): 672–74.

Husk, G., and D. Waxman. 2004. "Using Data from Hospital Information Systems to Improve Emergency Department Care." *Society for Academic Emergency Medicine* 11 (11): 1237–44.

Langley, G. J., K. M. Nolan, T. W. Nolan, C. L. Norman, and L. P. Provost. 1996. *The Improvement Guide: A Practical Approach to Enhancing Organizational Performance.* San Francisco: Jossey-Bass Publishers.

Lewandrowski, K. 2004. "How the Clinical Laboratory and the Emergency Department Can Work Together to Move Patients Through Quickly." *Clinical Leadership and Management Review* 18 (3): 155–59.

Liew, D., and M. P. Kennedy. 2003. "Emergency Department Length of Stay Independently Predicts Inpatient Length of Stay." *Medical Journal of Australia* 179 (10): 516–17.

Wilson, M., and K. Nguyen, 2004. "Bursting at the Seams: Improving Patient Flow to Help America's Emergency Departments." Urgent Matters [Online whitepaper; retrieved 9/17/05.] www.urgentmatters.org/pdf/ UM_WhitePaper_BurstingAtTheSeams.pdf .

CHAPTER 6

Toolkit:
Strategies for a
Systems Approach

It is hard to push with a rope—pulling works better.

— Irish proverb

MANAGING PATIENT FLOW throughout healthcare systems is an ever-changing combination of art and science, using business tools, metrics, and technology to improve the healthcare experience for patients, staff, and administrators. Much of this work focuses on changing the relationships among the various microsystems (the ED, surgery, the PACU, the ICU, the catheterization lab, and so on) that comprise the hospital and healthcare community—that is, creating a system that pulls patients through the system in an orderly, logical, and predictable progression.

Like the skier gliding downhill, the patient should move easily from one service to another in the hospital, using the natural gravity or "pull" of the system. Providers in the ED should not be beating on the ICU doors to admit a critical patient; the cardiac unit should not be holding a ready-to-discharge patient for hours because they are waiting for pharmacy to send needed medication; discharge services should not be holding a patient all afternoon while she is waiting for a ride. With service innovations and metrics, you can predict and plan daily routines so that service providers can be proactive rather than reactive. The ICU knows about how many people will need to come in on a given day and can say, "Who may be ready to go to step-down this afternoon?"

Pharmacy can say, "Who is leaving cardiac care tomorrow and what will they need?"

Discharge can say, "You will be discharged tomorrow at 3 p.m. if all goes as planned. How can we help ensure that your family will be here then?" A pull system enables the valves in the flow system to remain open.

FLOW IN THE EMERGENCY DEPARTMENT

Because the ED is a main point of entry into the healthcare system—a main valve—flow from the ED into the hospital units critically affects the flow of the healthcare system as a whole. Therefore, to make real improvements in flow, a high-performance ED must have processes that are synchronized with those in the other parts of the hospital.

Because the ED has long served as the hospital's front door for many patients, the opportunities for improvement in service operations are perhaps more richly developed here than anywhere else in the healthcare system ("You seldom get a second chance to make a first impression")—or perhaps creative efforts and research have been focused on the ED because necessity is the mother of invention. Although significant and profound innovations in patient flow have been made in clinic and outpatient settings (see the IHI web site on the open access model for outpatient clinics and services and patient flow through acute care settings), the toolkit outlined in this chapter may appear to at times focus on initiating change, refinement, and improvement in patient flow in the ED. However, consider not only the techniques but also the principles to see that much of this material can be adapted to various inpatient units.

As the number of ED visits has risen and the number of hospital beds and ED nurses has fallen in the United States, many EDs have become overcrowded and chaotic. Ironically, this circumstance-induced dysfunction has come to be accepted as the norm. Hospital administrators, as well as patients, often expect the interminable unpleasant wait and surly ED service. They throw up their hands and say, in effect, "That's just the way it is in the ED." On the caregivers' side, we often see learned helplessness and/or cynicism: the problems are so entrenched that staff do not feel there is any hope of making a difference, so they give up or move on. The consequent indifference to improving conditions exacerbates the problem.

Because ED dysfunction has come to be accepted as the norm, we often no longer even recognize it. What does a dysfunctional department look like? The environment is often unpleasant, with spaces that are cramped and cluttered. A rickety side table may hold a stack of dog-eared, four-year-old *People* magazines and a *Guideposts* or two. The plastic plants that are way past needing replacement indicate that hospital staff do not really care what the room looks like or how it makes the people who use it feel. They have forgotten that for at least 50 percent (in some hospitals, as many as 70 percent) of their patients and their families, this is the hospital's front door. Typically, this ED has inadequate staff, and frustrated, disgruntled nurses and physicians. Lab and radiology TATs stretch to hours, especially during peak loads. Long waits create a lobby stacked with sick and injured patients and families who are often themselves frustrated and angry. Is this where you want to work? Think about this: if you wouldn't want to work here—if this is an environment where you can't fulfill your personal and professional mission of delivering superb healthcare—why would you or anyone want to come here as a patient?

Imagine, on the other hand, an emergency visit that is a pleasing or at least a satisfying experience for your patients. The waiting room is comfortable, with a receptionist who is friendly and eager to greet the patients, directing them to the Fast Track area if they have a child with an ear infection, have a sprained ankle, or have run out of medicine, for example. If patients must wait because a room is not available, they have adequate lighting, adequate space, adequate amenities, and appropriate reading material. A play area is available for young children, with books and upbeat videos. Patients are kept informed about the course of their stay throughout the emergency visit. Relatives are kept informed when patients are being treated or moved. Providers give patients and families business cards with contact information. The treatment area is spacious and comfortable, with room for the patient and room for storage and placement of supplies and equipment. The staff is pleasant and concerned, delivering the kind of quality care that they would like to deliver. A fantasy? Not at all.

Contrary to popular belief, chaos and dysfunction are not "the way it is" in EDs. All over the country, EDs have awakened to the fact that patients are not going to go away and that it is counterproductive to want them to. EDs are vital to the hospital business that provides the livelihood for healthcare workers. Ponder this: what would things look like if 50 percent of your admissions suddenly disappeared? Discouraging use of the ED is like saying, "I have a restaurant but I don't want you to eat here." In accepting or even tacitly encouraging a culture of chaos in the ED, we have lost our perspective. We need to change how we do things to better use resources and adapt systems to meet patient needs.

Hospitals that want to remain competitive, therefore, are learning to adapt their systems to attract and better serve the ED customer. They borrow ideas from the service industry to improve the environment and the service. Overlook Hospital in Summit, New Jersey, for example, has doubled its ED space in a renovation that included installation of a skylight and a water wall. The Medical University of Charleston's Trident Medical Center in South Carolina has private ED rooms and a children's play area. Inova Fairfax Hospital in Virginia has trained physicians and nurses on how to soothe patients who are upset about wait times. These healthcare systems all recognize the value of the ED as a key player in hospital-wide flow.

So what does it take to create a high-performance ED that connects effectively to the healthcare system as a whole? In Chapter 4 we discussed the importance of talented and committed leadership. For that leadership to be effective, a vision or a model is needed for the

Figure 6.1. Service Cycles and Subcycles in the ED

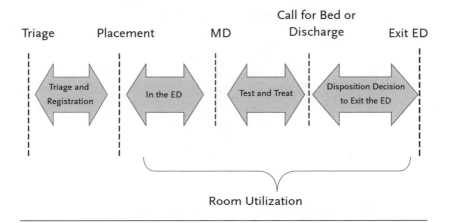

ED. Is the ED a key part of your hospital mission? Is it a centerpiece for the kind of service you deliver? Once you have decided what you want your ED to be like, formulate a strategy and look at the science around operations, patient safety, and patient service. The ED, with its activity cycles and subcycles, offers many opportunities for innovation and improvement in processes and service (Figure 6.1). Consider local ideas, import change concepts or change packages, and then be sure that people in the department have the skills to execute the change process. As author Jim Collins (2001) advises, "Get the right people on the bus."

One important concept is ensuring that each flow strategy is assessed according to the guiding vision of the organization. For example, Thom Mayer and other leaders at BestPractices, Inc., an emergency physician leadership and staffing company, assess all flow initiatives according to what they describe as "Rule #1, Rule #2":

- Rule #1: Is it good for the patient?
- Rule #2: Is it good for the people who take care of the patient?

Figure 6.2. Quality Improvement, Information Technology, and Clinical Medicine

Quality Improvement
- Flow teams
- System approach

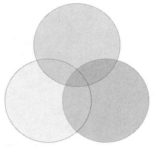

Information Technology
- Metric-based management
- Real-time data

Clinical Medicine
- Evidence-based guidelines
- Patient safety iniatives

Thus, if the flow initiative is good for the patient (Rule #1) and good for those who care for the patient (Rule #2), it is probably going to be a reasonable approach.

THE FLOW TOOLKIT

Following are the top strategies for improving flow that are essential for the flow improvement toolkit. They are derived from all the areas explored in this book: service, technology, and processes. Some of the most exciting innovations will likely take place where the domains of quality improvement, information technology, and clinical medicine overlap (Figure 6.2). Some apply mostly or only to the ED, and some only to the inpatient units, but all are essential to smoothing flow and improving service quality for patients and staff. Each of the flow initiatives can be evaluated according to a matrix that uses all of these elements of flow, the Flow Master Matrix (Figure 6.3).

The Flow Master Matrix simply takes the five features of flow defined in Chapter 1 and provides a structure through which to assess the likely impact of any flow initiative, including those concepts from the toolkit offered here or any other that your team develops. To recap, the five features of flow are as follows:

1. Improved efficiency and reduced cycle times
2. Reduced variation, increased predictability, improved forecasting
3. Systems thinking
   - Systems transitions
   - Alignment of incentives
4. Empowered providers exceeding expectations
5. Demand-capacity management

Each of the five features of flow is assessed by a Likert scale (1 to 5), estimating the tools' likely impact on each of the areas in the hospital. Based on the total score, leaders can make a reasoned assessment of the likelihood that the initiative will succeed in improving healthcare flow.

Based on the total score, projects receive a:

- Green Light (high impact on flow—go!)
- Yellow Light (medium impact on flow—go with caution, check strategic and tactical flow)
- Red Light (minimal flow impact—reconsider carefully)

Green light programs can be pursued enthusiastically, but of course with a focus on process and metrics to measure results. Yellow light projects should often be pursued, if the strategic and tactical fit is good and if metrics can be used to measure success. If a flow initiative has a red light score after careful consideration by multiple stakeholders, then the initiative should be reconsidered carefully before deciding to proceed. Moreover, each flow initiative should continue to be assessed and reassessed, driven by data over the course

Figure 6.3. The Flow Master Matrix™

Score	Rating	Result
≥20	Green Light	High impact on flow
14–19	Yellow Light	Medium impact on flow Check strategic/tactical fit
≤14	Red Light	Minimal flow impact Reconsider carefully

Flow Initiative

5 Flow Factors	Fast Track	Advanced Time	Adopt-a-Boarder	Hospitalists	Surgical Scheduling
1. Reduce cycle time					
2. Reduce variation, improve predictability, increase forecasting					
3. Systems thinking • Systems transitions • Alignment of incentives					
4. Empowerment/ Exceeding expectations					
5. Demand-capacity management					

Rank each potential total initiative on a Likert scale (1–5). For systems thinking (#3), rank both systems transitions and alignment of incentives and divide by two for the score of the project. Finally, cost and return on investment, as well as the difficulty of change management, should be considered in each flow initiative. Because of the wide variation in these areas, each must be addressed on a local level. To see how this works, the evaluation of several flow toolkit items are discussed as innovations for the hospital using the matrix.

Emergency Department Fast Track

> When I use a word, it means precisely what I choose it to mean.
> —Lewis Carroll, *Through the Looking Glass*

"Fast Track" is a term that is widely used, but means different things to different people in different settings. As we mentioned before, "Fast Track" is usually a noun—a place in the ED where patients with minor illnesses and injuries are evaluated and treated. That is the sense in which we use the term here. But it can also be a verb—we "fast track" numerous patients according to a protocol-driven, evidence-guided, and therefore expedited approach. Trauma and chest pain patients are good examples of patients who are "fast tracked" in every good ED.

Patients with simple or discrete problems should be processed through a part of the ED where it is easy to handle simple problems: the Fast Track. Resources can be matched to service needs. Imagine that after a busy day at work, you stop by the supermarket. You pick up a bag of chips, a bottle of aspirin, and a Coke. You go to the checkout line. You find yourself behind the customer with four kids who is doing his weekly grocery shopping. You know that you don't need much time at the register. But in a first in, first out system, you are going to be waiting in line for a long time. In engineering terms, anytime a first in, first out system is applied at high-volume processing points, easy-to-process items slow down as they wait in queue.

Many patients come into the ED knowing that all they need is a prescription, an x-ray, or a medical opinion. They don't need to stack up behind the patient with congestive heart failure, chronic obstructive pulmonary disease, or AIDS who requires an extensive and lengthy diagnostic workup and treatment. In a first in, first out system, unless there is a way to process those patients with simple needs, they will wait. The Fast Track is not a safety valve that is used just for overflow, but a separate product line for a distinct set of patients. Fast Track is a verb, not a noun, and the strategies that make it work can be applied to any incoming patient stream for which it makes sense.

The Fast Track needs space, staff and supplies, entry criteria, and protocols. An effective and efficient Fast Track can care for patients in a timely manner. Most EDs underutilize the Fast Track. An ED with a census of over 40,000 visits a year may have a three- or four-bed Fast Track, often a makeshift three or four beds, at that. While this limited level of commitment will improve care for a limited number of patients, it misses the primary point of having a Fast Track: to enable an ED to quickly identify patients with limited diagnostic and therapeutic needs and expedite the care of those patients. Most EDs can see 30 to 40 percent of patients in the Fast Track, and some, depending on the demographics, may be able to care for as many as 50 percent of patients through the Fast Track.

Using the strategy of demand-capacity management, the Fast Track should gear its hours of operation toward statistically analyzed and assessed arrival times for patients with a core group of Fast Track diagnoses and complaints. The hourly capacity of the Fast Track, in terms of space and staff, should be based on the hourly demand (or arrival) of Fast-Track-eligible patients. Most EDs operate their Fast Track units from mid or late morning to approximately 11 p.m. However, if performance improvement data indicate the need for a broader window for Fast Track hours, it may be operated as many as 16 to 24 hours per day, again based on a careful analysis of performance improvement and patient flow data. At Nash Health Systems in North Carolina, for example, Fast Track hours were 11 a.m. to 11 p.m. When the data were tracked, however, peak demand was found to be from 9 a.m. to 1 a.m. The Fast Track was closed during four hours of peak demand. The Fast Track hours were then extended, which raised the service quality and improved flow for all patients in the ED. If the data show that the patients start clustering or bottlenecking at 10 a.m., then the Fast Track should open before this happens, upstream of the service bottleneck. Track your data and match your operations to meet the need. Match your service capacity to your service demand.

Unfortunately, many EDs open their Fast Track in the afternoon hours, when the queue is already quite long, and subsequently end up playing "catch up" throughout the rest of the day. This is a major irritant to clinical staff, patients, and families—the term "Fast Track" seems very much an irony. Remember the principles involved here are as follows:

- "Fast Track" is a verb and not a noun.
- Fast Track capacity should match the demand for Fast Track services.

These Fast Track concepts apply to incoming patient streams at other points of entry in the healthcare system, not just to the ED. For inpatient units, patients can be segmented by looking at such markers as the following:

- patient acuity (triage levels);
- chief complaint (e.g., chest pain, stroke, congestive heart failure, asthma, orthopedics); and
- need for services (x-ray or no x-ray, lab or no lab, gurney or no gurney).

While experience indicates that Fast Track is successful, the Flow Master Matrix analysis validates this concept (Figure 6.4).

Reduced Cycle Time
Given the proper scope and resources dedicated to a Fast Track, most EDs can operate with a goal of 90 percent of patients being seen in 60

Figure 6.4. Flow Master Matrix: Fast Track

Flow Master Elements		Score
1.	Reduced cycle time	4–5
2.	Variation, prediction, forecasting	4–5
3.	Systems approach	3–4
	a) Service transitions	4–4
	b) Alignment of incentives	3–4
4.	Empowered expectations	4–5
5.	Demand-capacity management	5
		20–24
		GREEN LIGHT

minutes or less (there are always some patients who are triaged to Fast Track and who turn out to have a more complicated diagnosis, which largely accounts for the 10 percent that are seen in over 60 minutes). For many EDs, the reduction in cycle time is extremely dramatic when sufficient resources (space, staff, and services) are dedicated to the Fast Track. Depending on the appropriate triage protocols, resources, commitment, and changes driven by continuous process improvement or "tweaks" to the program, Fast Tracks typically score either a four or a five on reduced cycle time.

Reduced Variation, Improved Prediction, Improved Forecasting

Because Fast Tracks deal with a limited scope of illnesses and injuries, they dramatically reduce variation, especially if data are used to predict and forecast needs in the Fast Track area. Again, depending on the proper utilization of ongoing process- and performance-improvement tools, Fast Tracks score a solid four or five in this category.

Systems Thinking: Service Transitions and Alignment of Incentives

Despite the fact that the Fast Track deals with patients who almost exclusively will be treated and released from the ED, from a systems-thinking perspective, improved service transitions and alignment of incentives are still needed. Nearly 50 percent of Fast Track patients need either lab or x-ray services. Within the Fast Track itself, physicians, nurses, and all support personnel have very clearly aligned incentives and specific goals for moving patients through as expeditiously as possible. For this reason, Fast Tracks score either a three or four in this category, depending on the level of commitment and operational concerns at a local level.

Demand-Capacity Management

Guided by the appropriate process improvement data geared toward the Fast Track diagnostic group, this concept scores a solid five if appropriate resources (including staff, space, systems, and support services) are brought to bear at maximum peak flow times. Indeed, demand capacity management is at the heart of the Fast Track concept.

Empowered Expectations

Precisely because the physicians, nurses, and other staff in the Fast Track are geared toward meeting the needs of low-acuity, low-technical-intensity patients, they are capable of delivering a very high level of service when appropriately empowered to meet and exceed patient expectations. If ED leadership is supportive, Fast Tracks score a solid four or five in this area.

The Fast Track is an essential patient flow tool, as both observation and the matrix show. Without a Fast Track, the very patients who are easiest to treat in the ED and who require the least amount of resources—the minor to moderate medical and surgical emergencies—are the ones who are forced to wait the longest. These are the patients who will have the greatest impact on the community. By ramping up resources and time allocated to the Fast Track, an ED is guaranteed to see improvement in throughput.

The flow sheet and matrix are useful tools for predicting and measuring progress as you try the other flow ideas presented in this chapter. Tracking your data and using rapid-cycle testing will help you get started.

THE FLOW TEAM

Because flow is a property of the healthcare system as a whole, improving patient flow requires a systems approach. As we have already established, nobody wins when departments function as separate silos, and a flow problem in the ED must be seen from the broader perspective of the institution. Therefore, the flow team requires participation from staff leaders both inside and outside the ED (see Figure 4.2). First, the patient flow coordinator (the charge nurse in a previous life) must watch the big picture of patient flow in the ED and monitor whatever real-time data feeds are available. The patient flow coordinator should not just recognize flow problems but also needs to anticipate them. Second, the bed "czar" (or czarina) monitors flow from the inpatient side to keep track of bed turns and patient movement throughout the system. When a patient leaves the ICU, another patient should be swiftly brought to that bed. In fact, the ICU staff should be "pulling" that next patient into the ICU. Using data, the OR manager can smooth the surgical schedule, eliminating as much unnecessary variation as possible to facilitate flow from and through other acute care settings like the ED.

Back in the department, the ED physicians, charge nurses, registration team members, and technologists make board rounds to assess how the department functions at times of stress and to look for real-time process changes to facilitate flow. While the terms for this process may vary—"board rounds," "patient flow rounds," "bed board rounds"—the concept or model can and should be used at both the hospital (system) and unit (microsystem) level.

A key point is that the patient flow team (either the formal or informal team) consists of critical personnel both in and outside the ED, working together and using a systems approach to better benefit the patients and those who serve them.

Figure 6.5. Integrated Tracking System

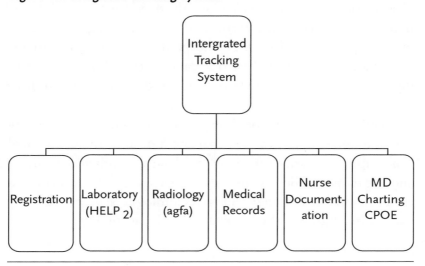

THE FLOW DASHBOARD:
INFORMATION TECHNOLOGY AND FLOW

Dashboard technology has been used in business and industry for many years and provides an integral tool for managing flow. In the most progressive models, data feeds from all aspects of operations cue the tracking system when process delays are occurring. This integrated system pulls together all of the islands of information relevant to the ED patient visit or to the patient care unit being monitored (Figure 6.5).

Frontline practitioners can then try to address these bottlenecks in real time by altering operations to accommodate demand. The dashboards are the tools that enable this important paradigm shift from retrospective to real-time process improvement. For instance, at one hospital with a homegrown tracking system with dashboards, when the radiology TAT exceeds one hour or more than five patients are waiting for x-rays, either backup staff are called in or the patients are taken to the main x-ray department to speed up the radiology operations. This type of contingency plan allows the department to build elasticity into its service operations and to use existing resources to match capacity to demand. The hospital can also save all patient-care-related data in a database (the data mart) for future data mining efforts to both analyze bottlenecks and improve patient flow forecasting.

While the old whiteboard may continue to serve as a meeting site (the water cooler) in the department or unit, the whiteboard is not up to the task of tracking the details of individual patient and departmental flow. Currently 50 percent of EDs have moved to electronic technology. This technology lags considerably behind this figure at the hospital and/or inpatient unit level.

ADVANCED TRIAGE PROTOCOLS

The Fast Track concept focuses on diverting patients with minor illnesses or injuries to a specific area of the ED with dedicated resources, but what happens when "demand" exceeds "supply"—in other words, when the system has more patients to be seen than capacity to see them? When the rooms are full and the queue is growing, what do you do?

Over 12 years ago, physicians and nurses at Inova Fairfax Hospital looked at this problem and came up with a simple yet highly effective solution, which they termed "Advanced Triage–Advanced Initiatives™" or AT/AI™ for short. Simply stated, this approach involves taking standing physician orders for the triage nurses to use for patients with specified chief complaints, which allows initial care and treatment to begin prior to being assigned a room. Chief-complaint-based standardized order sets have been shown to improve throughput and decrease medical errors. Progressive EDs are developing them locally for their most common chief complaints. These triage protocols allow the staff to begin the diagnostic and therapeutic journey in advance of the physician seeing

Figure 6.6. Flow Master Matrix: Advanced Triage Protocols

Flow Master Elements		Score
1.	Reduced cycle time	4–5
2.	Variation, prediction, forecasting	4–5
3.	Systems approach	4–5
	a) Service transitions	4–5
	b) Alignment of incentives	4–5
4.	Empowered expectations	5
5.	Demand-capacity management	4
		21–24
		GREEN LIGHT

the patient. Nurses like them because they empower the staff to begin treating patients. For example, a patient comes in with an ankle sprain. The physician walks in after two hours and says, "You need an ankle x-ray." The patient says, "No kidding." The physician adds value to this process by interpreting the x-ray and formulating a therapeutic plan, not by deciding whether or not the x-ray is needed. X-ray protocols allow nurses to order x-rays, a process that can save a lot in throughput time and patient satisfaction as the physician sees the patient and the x-ray simultaneously. These protocols are also particularly useful in the management of pain. By expediting pain control, the healthcare team improves both customer service and patient satisfaction.

These protocols must be collaboratively designed, implemented by effective inservices, and guided on an ongoing basis by process improvement data. However, once these conditions are met, the Flow Master Matrix score indicates that this is a highly effective flow strategy. Using the Flow Master Matrix, advanced triage protocols (Figure 6.6) typically score a 21 to 24, indicating a clear green light flow strategy.

Indeed, when the Health Care Advisory Board assessed the concept of advanced triage protocols, it was given a grade of "B+." In addition, in the authors' experience, triage nurses, primary care nurses, emergency physicians, and, most importantly, patients find this change to be effective for patient satisfaction, employee satisfaction, reduced turnaround time, and patient safety. For all of these reasons, "Advanced Triage—Advanced Initiatives" is a concept that most EDs should use at times when rooms are not available for patients to be seen. It is extremely important, both for patient satisfaction and for compliance with Joint Commission protocols, that some element of effective pain management is built within the advanced triage protocols.

DIRECT-TO-ROOM/TRIAGE BYPASS

Consider the following story:

> I was traveling recently and was dismayed when I arrived at the airline ticket counter to find that the "cattle gates" were up, through which you had to walk to speak to the ticket agent. But this was my lucky day—there was no one in line, so I stepped around the gate and walked directly up to the ticket agent.
>
> She said, "Sir, I'm sorry, but I've been instructed that I can't take care of people until they have gone through the line." I looked behind me just to recheck and said, "But … there is no line." She said firmly, "Sir, I'm sorry, but I can't take care of you until you walk through the line."
>
> I glanced around, wondered if I was on Candid Camera, and, being married, realized that I take direction extremely well. So I walked around the line, quickly taking a series of lefts and rights, and stood at the head of the "line."
>
> The ticket agent looked at me and said, "Next!"

This sounds like a silly story, doesn't it? Why should someone have to go through the "maze" when there is no one in line to begin with? But that's precisely what happens on a daily basis in EDs and for many elective admissions and surgeries. In other words, we have one process, assuming there will be a line, but not a second process for when there is no line. Consider this example:

> At 9 a.m. (which is typically a relatively slow time in the ED), five patients arrive at the triage area within several minutes of each other. At most EDs, each patient is triaged sequentially and then sent along to the next step in the process, registration, after which a room is assigned in the treatment area, often at the convenience of the staff. Each of the patients works her way through the "maze," and the last one waits until all of the previous ones have gone through this process.

This is a daily occurrence in EDs because we are focusing on a single process. However, at BestPractices, Inc., this process has been redefined during specific times of the day when rooms, nurses, and other personnel are available to see patients and yet multiple patients present to triage. The concept is known as either "direct-to-room" or "triage bypass." It takes the simple if perhaps obvious insight that, at that particular time, each of those patients will be seen in the same rooms, by the same nurses, by the same technicians, and by the same emergency physicians, regardless of what their triage category is. If these conditions are met (and they are met on a daily basis at predicted times of the day as demonstrated by process improvement efforts), then the patients are sent directly back to the room, where they can be registered through bedside registration and their care expedited, even though the actual triage process will occur by the nurse in the treatment area instead of at the triage desk. An alternative to this process is "mini-triage," in which a more focused triage evaluation occurs, after which the patient is sent directly to the room for bedside registration.

This strategy has much more impact on the ED nursing staff than on the emergency physicians, and therefore appropriate planning and buy-in must occur from nursing for the strategy to be effective. In effect, the locus of control moves from the charge nurse in the typical ED process to the triage nurse in a direct-to-room scenario. As

Figure 6.7. Flow Master Matrix: Direct-to-Room/Triage Bypass

Flow Master Elements		Score
1.	Reduced cycle time	5
2.	Variation, prediction, forecasting	4–5
3.	Systems approach	4
	a) Service transitions	4
	b) Alignment of incentives	4
4.	Empowered expectations	4
5.	Demand-capacity management	5
		22–23
		GREEN LIGHT

Figure 6.7 shows, direct-to-room/triage bypass is an effective strategy, but is not as highly rated as Fast Track or advanced triage for the following reasons.

First, this strategy is effective only at times of the day when more rooms are available than there are patients to be seen. These times can be reasonably predicted by appropriate use of process improvement data. For many overcrowded EDs, this constitutes a relatively small percentage (less than 25 percent) of the time during the typical day. Second, using this strategy also assumes that bedside registration is available and functions at a high level, which should be a reasonable expectation for any ED dedicated to patient flow. Third, the strategy further requires, at least relatively, that there be a single treatment area open at the time that triage bypass is used. In other words, if there are multiple treatment areas (critical care, urgent care, pediatric care), triage bypass is slightly more complicated, since determination must be made with regard to which treatment area patients should be sent. Finally, as indicated previously, this is a change in the locus of control in the ED, and it therefore requires somewhat more significant change management efforts. Nonetheless, direct-to-room/triage bypass scores 22–23 on the Flow Master Matrix, which indicates that this is a green light concept. It deserves careful consideration of obstacles, but implementation thereafter.

TRIAGE ALTERNATIVES

From Virginia to Australia, traditional triage is being challenged. Triage is often a bottleneck to patient flow because the world must funnel through this entity to be treated, but is it always a necessary or useful bottleneck? One variation on traditional triage is "physician (or mid-level) triage," or having the clinician in triage, which expedites flow by getting the doctor and the patient together sooner. An innovative variation is Thom Mayer's "team triage." In this design, the entire team—doctor, nurse, and technicians—sees the patient and begins to work with the patient in parallel. Another variation being trialed is the so-called (for lack of a more cogent term) triage to the diagnostic waiting room. In this setting the patient is triaged back to the waiting room, where a tracking board is visible for patients to track their own progress. Further, family members help care for patients in the diagnostic waiting room.

These alternative triage structures work even better when the ED physician is empowered to admit patients. Sometimes it takes several hours to get attending physicians to see patients. Three separate studies have looked at the ability of an experienced ED physician to predict the need for admission when she walks out of a patient's room—without the benefit of lab tests or studies, and with an old chart. On average, 90 percent of the time the emergency physician knows when a patient needs to be admitted. So why does she wait two to three hours to get a bed? Because the wait is customary, and part of the culture. Changing the culture to empower the ED physician to make admission decisions keeps the flow moving.

Team triage, which was developed at Inova Fairfax Hospital's department of emergency medicine, recognizes that bottlenecks occur at predictable times and simply places a team comprising an emergency physician, nurse, registrar, scribe, and technician to begin treatment at the triage area. The results from the program have been dramatic, since nearly a third of patients can be evaluated and their treatment completed in this step. Many patients are admitted to the hospital without ever getting into a treatment room, implying that their care

Figure 6.8. Flow Master Matrix: Team Triage

Flow Master Elements		Score
1.	Reduced cycle time	4
2.	Variation, prediction, forecasting	4–5
3.	Systems approach	5
	a) Service transitions	5
	b) Alignment of incentives	5
4.	Empowered expectations	5
5.	Demand-capacity management	5
		23–24
		GREEN LIGHT

was actually completed in the ED prior to the time they would have been placed in a room. Not surprisingly, turnaround time, patient satisfaction, employee satisfaction, and profitability are all extremely high for this revolutionary concept. Team triage, according to the Flow Master Matrix, shows a score of 23 to 24, making it clearly a green light idea (Figure 6.8).

ADOPT-A-BOARDER/FULL CAPACITY PROTOCOL

The Adopt-a-Boarder program and the Full Capacity Protocol, the flow strategies implemented at Inova Fairfax and Stony Brook, are excellent strategies to use when, despite good flow initiatives, the ED gets overburdened. At these hospitals, as at countless others, a high rate of admission frequently resulted in the boarding of admitted patients in the ED hallways. The ED was constantly stressed by the clinical burdens of these admitted patients.

Adopt-a-Boarder and Full Capacity Protocol allow for the preferential boarding of admitted patients in inpatient hallways instead of the ED, decompressing the overcrowded area. Further, by involving other inpatient areas in the overcrowding problem, these initiatives foster new solutions and a new level of cooperation throughout the

Figure 6.9. Flow Master Matrix: Adopt-a-Boarder/Full Capacity Protocol

Flow Master Elements		Score
1.	Reduced cycle time	4
2.	Variation, prediction, forecasting	4
3.	Systems approach	3–4
	a) Service transitions	4
	b) Alignment of incentives	3
4.	Empowered expectations	4
5.	Demand-capacity management	4
		19–20
		YELLOW LIGHT

healthcare system. Facilitated discharges, improved thallium stress-testing turnarounds, inpatient bed expansions, and improved staffing ratios have all been offshoots of these innovations.

A completely unexpected positive outcome of the Adopt-a-Boarder approach was significantly reduced inpatient LOS, probably a result of patients getting specialty care earlier. Almost a full day of hospitalization was saved by moving the patients to inpatient unit hallways.

The Flow Master Matrix for Adopt-a-Boarder/Full Capacity Protocol (Figure 6.9) shows a score of 19 to 20, or yellow light. While this is a creative flow initiative, in many respects the goal is to prevent the need for Adopt-a-Boarder/Full Capacity Protocols. In other words, it is a great strategy but you do not want to have to use it!

CLINICAL DECISION UNITS

As the average ED census in the United States has risen over the past 20 years from 20,000 visits to 40,000 visits, so too have the different streams of patients coming into the ED. Initially, ED practitioners realized that ED patients could be segmented according to acuity and diagnostic complexity. The Fast Track was developed to accommodate the lower-acuity patients whose care could

Figure 6.10. Complexity of Patient Care with Age

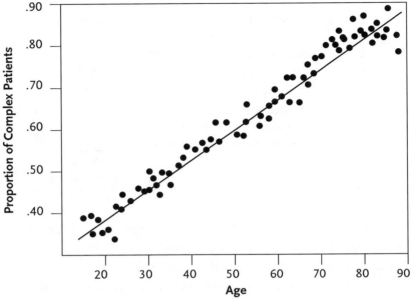

Source: Emergency Medicine Australasia. Used with permission.

be expedited in the ED. Following that innovation, the observation unit was developed to accommodate patients who needed 24 hours or less of hospitalization, and observation medicine took off under the emergency medicine domain. As the complexity of patients' care increases with increasing age (Figure 6.10), so does the time required to evaluate these patients in the ED.

CT scans of the abdomen with contrast, MRI scans, Doppler, and other vascular studies are becoming common diagnostic adjuncts in the ED, but they take time. Many leaders in emergency medicine are realizing the need for patients to remain in the ED for six to eight hours while tests are completed. This stream of patients typically has a high diagnostic intensity in the beginning of the ED visit, but subsequently needs fewer resources. These patients are being clustered in areas of the ED dubbed "clinical decision units." This innovation allows for patients to be maximally cared for at the outset, but for resources to be pulled back later in the ED visit.

Leadership for Smooth Patient Flow

Figure 6.11. Flow Master Matrix: Clinical Decision Units

Flow Master Elements		Score
1.	Reduced cycle time	4–5
2.	Variation, prediction, forecasting	4
3.	Systems approach	5
	a) Service transitions	5
	b) Alignment of incentives	3–4
4.	Empowered expectations	4
5.	Demand-capacity management	5
		22–23
		GREEN LIGHT

Clinical decision units score a solid 22 to 23 in the Flow Master Matrix (Figure 6.11) and should be used in most healthcare systems.

RAPID RESPONSE TEAMS

Rapid Response Teams are a relatively recent intervention. These teams were pioneered in Australia, where they are known as medical emergency teams. A Rapid Response Team brings critical care expertise and skills to the patient's bedside. A clinical SWAT team responds to a call from a floor nurse made when a patient's condition deteriorates in specific ways. Most programs involve a set of criteria or "triggers" to initiate the call. The Rapid Response Team is typically composed of an experienced critical care nurse and a respiratory therapist, and may include a physician or a mid-level practitioner. The goal (and the documented result) is to get to patients before they start a downward clinical spiral from which there may be no pulling up. These teams have been shown to have a significant impact on patient safety and mortality (Figure 6.12), as well as on patient flow. In addition to the lives saved, ICU utilization and non-critical care bed utilization are dramatically conserved or improved. In addition, emergency physicians and nurses are less likely to get pulled out of the ED to

Figure 6.12. Rapid Response Team Results

Measure	Before Rapid Response Team	After Rapid Response Team	Relative Risk Reduction
No. of cardiac arrests	63	22	65% ($p = .001$)
Deaths from cardiac arrest	37	16	56% ($p = .005$)
No. of days in ICU post arrest	163	33	80% ($p = .001$)
No. of days in hospital post arrest	1363	159	88% ($p = .001$)
Inpatient deaths	302	222	25% ($p = .004$)

Source: Table adapted from Bellomo R., et al. 2003. "A Prospective Before and After Trial of a Medical Emergency Room." *Medical Journal of Australia.* 179 (6): 283. Used with permission.

respond to in-house clinical emergencies. (For a full discussion of this exciting intervention, visit the IHI's website, www.ihi.org.)

ELECTIVE SURGICAL FLOW

Elective surgical patients are a stream of patients who are in direct competition with ED patients for inpatient resources—in particular, beds. Some hospitals can predict when they will be on diversion each week as a function of the surgical schedule (when the heavy hitters operate). Although the surgical schedule is typically responsible for 30 percent of the inpatient admissions while the ED is responsible for 50 percent of admissions (or more), the OR schedule accounts for more than half

Figure 6.13. Flow Master Matrix: Elective Surgical Scheduling

Flow Master Elements		Score
1.	Reduced cycle time	5
2.	Variation, prediction, forecasting	4
3.	Systems approach	5
	• Service transitions	5
	• Alignment of incentives	5
4.	Empowered expectations	4
5.	Demand-capacity management	5
		23
		GREEN LIGHT

of the variation in that portion of the system. One way to accommodate this unnecessary variation is to manage it through scheduling. For instance, since Mondays are very high census days for the ED, some limitation of the OR schedule on Mondays would make sense in terms of ED flow. By studying variation in this area, the hospital can improve patient flow and better match capacity to demand. Another way is to follow the example of St. John's and set aside OR space and time for unscheduled surgeries—in effect scheduling them.

Figure 6.13 shows that elective surgical scheduling is a green light concept that should be much more widely used in healthcare systems.

BED MANAGEMENT: ELECTRONICS, THE BED CZAR, AND BED-AHEAD SYSTEM

What about the patients who need admitting? We have talked about overcrowding and boarding in the ED, but how do you keep this from happening? There are multiple incoming streams of patients into the hospital, and the ED actually competes with the surgical stream, the elective surgery stream, and the direct admission stream. In Figure 6.14, you can see the potential for bottlenecks and some of the strategies for smoothing patient flow. If your ED has an admission rate of 15 percent, and 30 percent of your available bed hours in the ED are used up by admissions, 30 percent of your productive capacity is spent on 15 percent, of your patients. The longer the patients wait, the less productive capacity you have. It is important to recognize this fact and compensate to prevent backups that create delays.

In the past, bed management meant a person, usually a nurse, in an isolated room, with a clipboard and a whiteboard. This person allocated beds on a first-come, first-served basis. However, hospitals are increasingly employing electronic bed-management systems, which often offer a data warehouse function that enables forecasting of patient flow and service demand using system data. This system also provides data transparency, with census information available throughout the institution. This keeps all staff apprised of where openings are among the hospital beds and eliminates the practice of bed hiding.

In addition to the technologic innovations associated with bed management, the human innovation of the bed czar functions in tandem with technology. This individual, bringing a wealth of understanding of the details of the bed allocation process, is empowered to control and manage bed allocation and resources, particularly in the critical service areas of housekeeping and patient transport.

Many hospitals have incorporated the use of patient flow board rounds and multidisciplinary rounds to foster improvements in information management, forecasting, and facilitating patient flow. Whenever possible, combining the information management capabilities of technology with the wisdom of the people who actually work in your healthcare system is a force multiplier.

As explored in detail in Chapter 4, patient flow in your healthcare system is highly predictable, as tracking and trending your data will show you. In this predictability lies the solution to many flow problems. For example, think of the daily quest for an inpatient bed.

Figure 6.14. Hospital-wide Patent Flow Streams

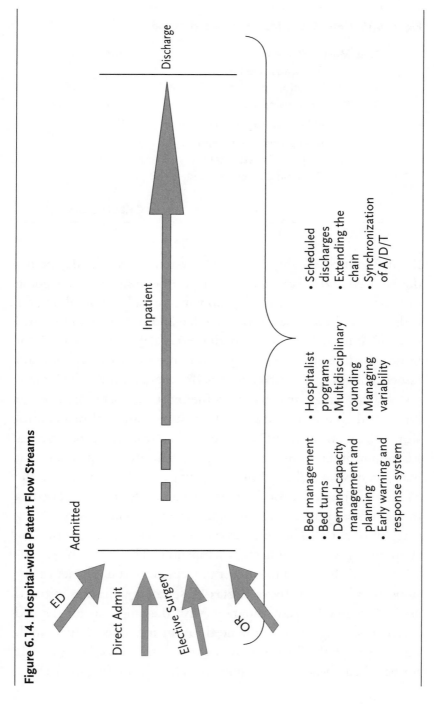

ED

Direct Admit

Elective Surgery

OR

Admitted

Inpatient

Discharge

- Bed management
- Bed turns
- Demand-capacity management and planning
- Early warning and response system

- Hospitalist programs
- Multidisciplinary rounding
- Managing variability

- Scheduled discharges
- Extending the chain
- Synchronization of A/D/T

Figure 6.15. Flow Master Matrix: Be-a-Bed-Ahead

Flow Master Elements		Score
1.	Reduced cycle time	5
2.	Variation, prediction, forecasting	5
3.	Systems approach	4–5
	a) Service transitions	4
	b) Alignment of incentives	5
4.	Empowered expectations	4
5.	Demand-capacity management	5
		23–24
		GREEN LIGHT

If you admitted roughly 18 patients yesterday and the day before that and every day last year and the year before that, you're going to need roughly 18 beds today. So why, instead of scrambling for beds each and every day, is the ED demand not factored into bed control? Why are you not preparing every day and every week for those 18 admissions per day (you can also calculate the variation associated with that average number)? To establish this bed-ahead system, the change that has been the most successful has been to center bed control in the ED. The czar or czarina of bed control works closely with the ED or reports directly to someone who has ED responsibilities. In the best systems, data are transparent—that is, everyone who makes a decision about patient flow that affects the ED or the unit under consideration has access to the necessary data in real time; visual indicators signal when patient flow is getting sluggish or sticky. The clinical bed control leaders get out on "the shop floor" to see what is really happening. They have the experience, the wisdom, and the power to facilitate and implement solutions in real time. At Inova Fairfax Hospital, the idea was initiated as the "be-a-bed-ahead" program, with the emphasis on the bed czar(ina) staying ahead of the need for inpatient beds, thus avoiding delays and the formation of a queue. The Flow Master Matrix for be-a-bed-ahead shows a solid green light score (Figure 6.15).

EXPRESS ADMISSION UNITS

Recognizing that bottlenecks frequently occur at the point of transfer, healthcare systems are turning to the concept of express admission units. In many EDs, the time from the decision to admit to obtaining admission orders averages one hour. Another 82 minutes pass before those orders are acted on. As many as 12 hours pass before the patient gets to the inpatient floor. Express units provide a physical space adjacent to the ED for patients to wait for their rooms to be ready and to complete the admission process, which is standardized and streamlined. These units are for patients who no longer need the therapeutic intensity of the main ED. Related innovations include a no-refusal policy for units accepting these admissions and the faxing of reports as opposed to time-consuming verbal reports. In addition, these units often have an admission SWAT team that includes housekeeping and transportation to facilitate the transfer of patients to inpatient units.

SCHEDULED AND STAGGERED DISCHARGES

While many hospitals still try to promote an "out by 11 a.m." discharge policy, others are adopting the concept of staggered scheduled discharges to smooth workload and reduce patient waits. In addition, the simple innovation of a small whiteboard in each patient's room that indicates the scheduled discharge time (a day in advance) along with what needs to happen before discharge (physical therapy consultation, dietary consultation, etc.) has had a positive effect on the process. With patients, family members, and staff all on the same page and understanding what needs to happen before discharge, the process is more smoothly implemented and timelines can be met. Facilities have created discharge lounges where patients can wait for transportation home so that beds may be cleaned. Some institutions are even providing van transportation home for patients for the sake of bed management. Certainly, institutions with robust discharge services are ahead of the game in terms of bed management and patient flow.

Figure 6.16. Hospitalists and Length of Stay

	66 hospitals with hospitalists	198 hospitals with no hospitalists
Average LOS	6.5 days	11.9 days
Occupancy rates	63%	55%
Operating expenses per discharge	$12,280	$11,685
Hospital return on investment	3.1%	(1%)

Source: Adapted in part from AcademyHealth. 2006. "Management, Organization, and Financing" [Online whitepaper; retrieved 9/26/06] http://www.academyhealth.org

HOSPITALISTS

In the late 1990s many internists began to favor a medical practice that existed only in the hospital, and the term "hospitalists" was coined. These physicians have an assertive and patient-flow-oriented practice style, are hospital-based, and embrace standardized protocols and technology. They are showing very positive results in terms of shortened LOS, higher return on investment, less resource utilization, and lower mortality rates (Figure 6.16). The hospitalists also have a positive impact on patient flow, in particular for patients coming from the ED into inpatient units. This is in part because they are based in the hospital—by expediting both diagnostic and therapeutic interventions, they can often facilitate a shortened LOS on the inpatient side, thereby increasing inpatient service capacity. Another benefit for the ED is that hospitalists tend to be responsive and timely when the ED calls.

Figure 6.17. Flow Master Matrix: Hospitalists

Flow Master Elements		Score
1.	Reduced cycle time	5
2.	Variation, prediction, forecasting	4–5
3.	Systems approach	5
	a) Service transitions	5
	b) Alignment of incentives	5
4.	Empowered expectations	4
5.	Demand-capacity management	5
		23–24
		GREEN LIGHT

The use of hospitalists, effectively guided by an evidence-based approach, can predictably result in a 1.5- to 2.5-day decrease in inpatient LOS and, not surprisingly, earns a Flow Master Matrix score of 23 to 24 (Figure 6.17). Green light!

CONCLUSION

While all the recommended tools and changes for improving patient flow have worked for many teams in many healthcare systems, there is no substitute for trying them out for yourself. Rapid cycle improvement strategies (see Chapter 5) can help you use these tools to improve flow in your own system. To achieve high performance, you need to formulate a focused strategic vision for what your healthcare system will be and to define the mission and performance standards of each of the individual clinical units. It is critical to see how each unit's services interact and integrate with the mission and services of all of the clinical units that form your healthcare system. Each of the key units, departments, and service lines has to be seen as a key customer of the other clinical service providers. If optimal flow is to be achieved, the need for staff, space, and information technology support must be carefully and frequently evaluated. Both the ED and the surgical service must be seen as key drivers of hospital-wide flow, margin, and clinical service. Because holding people and processes accountable for the desired level of performance is critical, performance objectives must be clear and transparent. High-level strategies include forecasting patient volume and complexity, matching capacity and demand, improving work flow processes, managing peak loads, decreasing variation, managing the waits, optimizing the work environment, designing appropriate facility layout and space, and shaping patient demand. As you work with the tools in this toolkit to transform patient flow in your healthcare system, you might draw inspiration from the observation of Peter Drucker: "The best way to predict the future is to create it."

References

Collins, J. 2001. *Good to Great*. New York: HarperCollins

Further Recommended Readings

Bazarian, J. J., S. M. Schneider, V. J. Newman, and J. Chodosh. 1996. "Do Admitted Patients Held in the Emergency Department Impact the Throughput of Treat and Release Patients?" *Academic Emergency Medicine* 3 (12): 1113–18.

Advisory Board. 2000. "Building the Clockwork Emergency Department: Best Practices for Eliminating Bottlenecks and Delays in the Emergency Department." Washington, DC: Advisory Board/HWorks.

Stony Brook University Hospital and Medical Center. 2001. "Full Capacity Protocol." [Online article; retrieved 9/26/06] www.viccellio.com/fullcapacity.htm.

Institute for Healthcare Improvement (IHI). 2003. "Optimizing Patient Flow: Moving Patients Smoothly Through Acute Care Settings." Boston: IHI. [Online white paper; retrieved 9/26/06] www.ihi.org/IHI/Results/WhitePapers/OptimizingPatientFlowMovingPatientsSmoothlyThroughAcuteCareSettings.htm.

Kelley, M. A. 1999. "The Hospitalist: A New Medical Specialty." *Annals of Internal Medicine* 130 (4): 373–75.

Wilson, M., and K. Nguyen, 2004. "Bursting at the Seams: Improving Patient Flow to Help America's Emergency Departments." Urgent Matters [Online whitepaper; retrieved 9/17/05.] www.urgentmatters.org/pdf/ UM_WhitePaper_BurstingAtTheSeams.pdf.

Afterword

As we conclude our exploration of patient flow, we need to make one more observation about the way things are done and why. Although this observation is not a benchmark for turnaround time, a patient benefit, a revenue source, or a service innovation, it is critical to all these things.

Consider this story about the space shuttle. It is not a tale of human error or system failures, of O-rings or foam insulation. The space shuttle is a marvelous invention. It is arguably the world's most advanced transportation system, capable of transporting human beings into space and bringing them back home again. It can do this over and over again. You have all seen pictures of the space shuttle on its launch pad. It looks like a futuristic airplane, nestled within two large haunches, ready to vault into space. Those two haunches are two big booster rockets attached to the sides of the main fuel tank. These are the solid rocket boosters, or SRBs for short.

The SRBs are made by Thiokol at its factory in Utah and are shipped by train from the factory to the launch site. The railroad line from the factory runs through a tunnel in the mountains. The SRBs, 12 feet in diameter, have to fit through that tunnel. The tunnel is slightly wider than the railroad track. The railroad tracks are 4 feet, 8.5 inches apart. Why this distance?

The first railroad lines were built by British expatriates, the same people who built the pre-railroad tramways. The people who built the first tramways used the same jigs and tools that they used for building horse-drawn wagons. The jigs for wagons set the wheels 4 feet, 8.5 inches apart because that was the width between the deep ruts on ancient long-distance British roads. The roads were built by Imperial Rome to accommodate the Roman war chariot. Roman chariots formed the initial ruts in the road, and everyone else followed in them. The wheels of the Roman war chariot were 4 feet, 8.5 inches apart to accommodate the width of two horses in harness.

So, the width of the solid booster rocket on the space shuttle, a modern engineering triumph, is determined by the width of a tunnel, which is set by the width of the railroad tracks, which is determined by the width between deep ruts in the British road made by Imperial Roman war chariots made wide enough to accommodate the width of two horses' behinds.

There may be a better way of constructing the system both for you and your patients. You don't have to keep doing things the same old way because it is the culture of your system, because everybody is comfortable with it, or because it is the way you've always done things. Sometimes the wheel, or in this case perhaps the road, *does* need to be reinvented. We must think beyond the systems we have inherited or that have evolved in ways that don't now work best for patients, healthcare workers, or administrators—and maybe never did.

> How can anyone doubt that a small group of dedicated people can change the world? Indeed, it is the only thing that ever has.
>
> —Margaret Mead

Using this book as a starting point, go back to your healthcare system and begin to change it. Ask yourself what you can do by next week. Change one process with one patient at one time. Then do it again. And again. And again. . . . When you find what works, make another change somewhere else. You have in hand the ideas to execute for a better way to deliver healthcare. With your will, you and your team can change the quality of life of those who come to you for help and healing—as well as the quality of your life and the lives of those with whom you work.

Definitions, Concepts, and Measures from Atlanta Summit Proceedings

1. General Definitions/Concepts for Emergency Department Performance

Emergency department (ED): A 24-hour location serving an unscheduled patient population with anticipated needs for emergency medical care.

Psychiatric ED: An ED developed and held out to the community as one that serves the unscheduled needs of patients with mental health conditions.

Arrival time: The time that the patient is first recognized and recorded by the ED system as requesting services in the department.

MD/LIP contact: The duration (in minutes) of first contact of the physician or licensed independent practitioner (LIP) with the patient to initiate the medical screening exam.

Decision to admit: The time at which the physician or LIP makes the decision to admit the patient; time of bed request may be used as a proxy.

Conversion time: The time at which the disposition is made for a patient to be admitted to the hospital as an inpatient or observation patient; or the time at which a patient is designated for observation within a clinical decision area of the ED.

Discharge time: The time of physical departure of a discharged patient from the ED treatment area.

Physician disposition time: The time from physician notification (generally an emergency physician, but may be medical staff physicians responsible for patients in the ED) that all results are available until disposition time.

Left ED: The time at which an admitted or transferred patient physically leaves the ED treatment area.

ED length of stay: The patient time in the ED with these markers:

- For admitted patients: Arrival time to conversion time
- For discharged patients: Arrival time to discharge time
- For transferred patients: Arrival time to transfer conversion time

Active acuity level: ESI is used for analysis of severity level of patients in the ED.

Boarding: The practice of holding patients in the ED for extended periods of time who have been directed for admission by a physician with admitting privileges. This process then contains certain elements of the admission process and ongoing patient care provided by ED staff members.

Boarded patient: An admitted patient for whom the time interval between decision to admit and physical departure of the patient from the ED treatment area (decision to left ED time) exceeds 120 minutes.

Daily boarding hours: The sum of boarded patient (see above) minutes in a 24-hour period. Divide total minutes by 60 to get hours of care provided by ED.

ED boarding load: This is a snapshot of the boarded patient load being cared for in an ED and an indirect marker for the complexity/severity of patients being held in the ED. Calculated as (number of admitted patients + observation patients + transferred patients)/total ED patient care spaces. It can be calculated at any time, and can be reported as a daily maximum value for a period of time.

Radiology turnaround time: The time from the placement of an order for a radiographic test until the time the results are returned.

Laboratory turnaround time: The time from the placement of an order for laboratory testing until the time the results are returned.

Decision to transfer: The time at which the physician or licensed independent practitioner makes the decision to transfer the patient to another facility; time of transfer request may be used as a proxy.

Transfer accepted: The time at which the patient is accepted for transfer by the receiving facility.

Pediatric patients: Age cut-off for performance measures to describe and monitor this population needs to be tied to the resources required to manage these patients. However, the group is recommending that key performance indicators be specific for the pediatric population in two age ranges:

- Age 0 to 2nd birthday
- Age 2 (2nd birthday) to 18th birthday

Pediatric EDs: Those EDs that are designed to serve the needs of a pediatric patient group. They should be defined as those EDs that see a patient population less than 18 years of age, for over 80 percent of the total volume. This designation should also be applied to portions of a multi-function ED that serve this targeted population.

2. Performance Measures/Time Measures

A. For discharged patients
- Door-to-doctor time: The time difference in minutes between arrival time and MD/LIP contact with the patient.
- Doctor-to-discharge time: The time difference in minutes

between MD/LIP contact with the patient and discharge time.

- ED LOS for discharged patients: The time difference in minutes between arrival time and discharge time.

B. For admitted patients:

- Door-to-doctor time: The time difference in minutes between arrival time and MD/LIP contact with the patient.
- Doctor-to-decision-to-admit time: The time difference in minutes between MD/LIP contact with the patient and the decision to admit.
- Decision-to-left-ED time: The time difference in minutes between the decision to admit and the physical departure of the patient from the ED treatment area.
- ED LOS for admitted patients: The time difference in minutes between arrival time and physical departure of the patient from the ED treatment area (sum of door-to-doctor time + doctor-to-decision-to-admit time + decision-to-left-ED time).
- Daily boarding hours: Sum of (decision-to-left-ED time – 120 minutes for each boarder)/60 for all boarders in a 24-hour period.

C. For transferred patients:

- Door-to-doctor time: The time difference in hours between arrival time and MD/LIP contact with the patient.
- Doctor-to-decision-to-transfer time: The time difference in hours between MD/LIP contact with the patient and the decision to transfer.
- Decision-to-transfer-time-to-transfer-accepted time: The time difference in hours between the decision to transfer the patient and the acceptance of the transfer.
- Transfer-accepted-to-left-ED time: The time difference in hours between the acceptance of transfer and the physical departure of the patient from the ED treatment area.
- ED LOS for transferred patients: The time difference in hours between arrival time and physical departure of the patient from the ED treatment area (sum of door-to-doctor time + doctor-to-decision to transfer time + decision-to-transfer time to transfer-accepted time + transfer-accepted-to-left-ED time).

3. Performance Measures/Proportion Measures

- Patients leaving before the medical screening exam (PLBM): This term refers to any patient who leaves the ED before initiation of the MSE. It is expressed as a rate of occurrences per 100 visits. Calculate the interval from the time the patient is recognized as an encounter in the ED to the time that the patient departed or the medical screening exam was initiated.

- Patients leaving after the medical screening exam (PLAM): This term refers to any patient who leaves the ED after the MSE, but before the provider-documented completion of treatment. It is expressed as a rate of occurrences per 100 visits. Calculate the interval from the time of the initiation of the MSE to the time that the patient departed.

- Patients who leave against medical advice (AMA): Any patient recognized by the institution and leaving after interaction with the ED staff but before the ED encounter is officially ended. This differs from PLAM in that it includes documentation of patient competence, discussion about risks and benefits, and completion of or refusal to complete documents confirming the intent to leave against the recommendation of medical care staff.

- Complaints: The definition should include all spontaneous concerns about service delivery in the ED, written or verbal, that are brought to the attention of ED leaders. Separate categories of service concerns should be those identified during a survey process or during the billing process. Complaints are typically counted as one complaint per communication and tracked in rates per 1,000 ED visits.

- Diversion: The reasons, methods, and responses to diversion of patients from the ED are felt to be widely variable and inconsistent. Regardless of the root cause, the reason an organization chooses to divert a patient from their ED is that in their judgment they are unable to provide appropriate services to that patient at that time. Quantifying the number of hours an ED maintains diversion status provides an indicator of frequency within that facility without indication of the cause or any way to compare to like facilities.

- ED diversion: ED diversion is an occurrence communicated to the community and Emergency Medical Services (EMS) providers indicating that resources in a hospital are compromised (due to relative shortages of available staff, equipment, or beds). It is a request for patients being transported by EMS to be taken to another hospital for service. There may be specific inclusion or exclusion of groups of patients, according to local EMS protocol. The diversion occurrences are tracked by the number of hours per time period when that request has been made.

4. Emergency Department Patient Flow

- Greater than six-hour stay: Capacity is reflected by patient length of stay, but the definition of "extended LOS" is arbitrary and not useful. In addition to monitoring minutes or hours of the patient stay, consider breaking LOS into fractiles. As with measures of flow and throughput, this group is recommending benchmarking to identify outliers and target root causes of barriers to throughput (see above.)

5. Census and Utilization Definitions and Markers

Definitions related to patient numbers:
- Patients per day
- Pediatric patients per day
- Patients per day stratified by code levels 1 through 5

Definitions related to patient acuity:
- Patients admitted per day
- Patients transferred per day
- High-acuity patients served. Physician-coded patients level 99284, 99285, and 99291

Definitions related to patient mix:
- Patient payer class divided into three groups:

1. Medicare patients
2. Medicaid plus self-pay
3. All patients with other payers

Defined elements of emergency service units:
- EKGs done per 100 patients seen
- Simple imaging procedures done per 100 patients seen
- CT or MRI scans done per 100 patients seen
- Trauma panel utilization per 100 patients seen
- Cardiac biomarker tests done per 100 patients seen
- Medication doses administered per 100 patients seen (eventually stratified by type of medication)

ED patient service areas:
- Designated "complete patient service care areas (CPCSAs)," defined as an area where complete health service can be delivered to patient and family for a specific period of time. Does not include hall areas, parking spaces, holding areas.
- ED crowding is defined as the number of hours (reported as a per-day element) where patient census exceeds designated CPSCAs.

ED service personnel:
- ED personnel should be defined as to their general function area, not the cost center they are assigned to. The reporting element is service hours per day.
- Physician or physician extender
- Resident physician
- Nursing and other direct patient care service
- Ancillary patient care service (radiology, lab, respiratory therapy, orthopedic technician)
- Ancillary non-patient service (clerical, maintenance, security, cleaning, IT, supply)

Patient care–specific factors designated by ED staff:
- Designated prisoners
- Designated patients presenting for care primarily related to mental health, chemical dependency, or both
- Designated patients for observation services in the ED (may

or may not be in an area designated as a clinical decision unit, but are undergoing lengthy evaluation or treatment services under the medical direction of the emergency physician, with the intent to finish that evaluation and treatment and be discharged out of the ED)

Source: Augustine, J.; Camago, C. A.; Reese, C.; and Welch, S. J. 2006. "Emergency Department Performance Measures and Benchmarking Summit," ACAD EMERG MED, Oct., Vol. 13, No. 10:1074-80.

Patient Flow Glossary

Adopt-a-Boarder (Full Capacity Protocol):   a process that involves placing patients in inpatient hallway beds as well as in ED hallway beds when the ED is crowded with admitted patients, thereby "sharing the pain" and improving patient satisfaction

Aim: A written, measurable, and time-sensitive statement of the expected results of an improvement process.

Bed board: A real-time or frequently updated visual display of unit capacity.

Bed czar: A person or persons responsible for managing patient admissions and transfers.

Bed huddle: A planning process for improving patient flow. Unit directors from across the hospital meet to review and act on admissions, discharges, and transfers within the hospital. The huddle provides an opportunity to review demand across the hospital, identify available beds, and manage transfers and discharges.

Bed turns: Number of times (to the nearest whole number) a bed is used by a patient, whether for admissions or for any type of observation.

Boarders: Patients who have been admitted to the hospital but do not have a bed in the intended admission or transfer unit due to lack of capacity.

Centralized bed authority: A person or persons responsible for all admissions and transfers.

Change concept: A general idea for changing a process. Change concepts are usually at a high level of abstraction, but evoke multiple ideas for specific processes. "Simplify," "reduce Handoffs," and "consider all parties as part of the same system" are all examples of change concepts.

Cycle or PDSA cycle: A structured trial of a process change. Drawn from the Shewhart cycle, this effort includes:

- Plan—a specific planning phase
- Do—a time to try the change and observe what happens
- Study—an analysis of the results of the trial
- Act—devising next steps based on the analysis

This PDSA cycle will naturally lead to the plan component of a subsequent cycle.

Discharge appointment: An appointment for patient discharge time based on predicted readiness of patient, estimated time to complete discharge processes, and availability of transportation.

Diversion: Hospitals functioning at or beyond capacity in the ED may divert, or not accept, urgent care patients transported by ambulance.

Downstream: Units accepting patients from other care areas are considered "downstream."

Early adopter: In the improvement process, the opinion leader within the organization who brings in new ideas from outside the organization, tries them, and uses positive results to persuade others in the organization to adopt the successful changes.

Early majority/late majority: The individuals in the organization who will adopt a change only after it is tested by an early adopter (early majority) or after the majority of the organization is already using the change (late majority).

Extending the chain: Working beyond the walls of the hospital, with resources in the community, to improve flow.

Fast Track: A process whereby patients with urgent conditions in the ED are separated from patients requiring a higher level of care. Fast track patients can be treated relatively quickly, reducing overall waiting time and improving flow of patients through the ED

Implementation: Taking a change and making it a permanent part of the system. A change may be tested first and then implemented throughout the organization.

Internal diversion: When patients are admitted or transferred to units without available beds, these patients are diverted to other units in the hospital.

IS: The information system in the organization, usually the computerized information system.

Key changes: The list of essential process changes that will help lead to breakthrough improvement, usually on literature and the experience of testing.

Measure: An indicator of change. Key measures should be focused, clarify your team's aim, and be reportable. A measure is used to track the delivery of proven interventions to patients and to monitor progress over time.

METs: Medical emergency team(s) include an ICU doctor on duty plus an intensive care nurse who respond to calls from nurses on other floors to assess the condition of a patient.

Model for improvement: An approach to process improvement, developed by Associates in Process Improvement, which helps teams accelerate the adoption of proven and effective changes.

Multidisciplinary rounds: A process utilized within and outside intensive care settings whereby a multidisciplinary team "rounds" on all patients to review clinical condition and establish daily goals.

Observation: The use of an inpatient bed for any amount of time when the patient is not formally admitted to the hospital.

Patient flow: The movement of patients through the acute care setting.

PDSA: Another name for a cycle (structured trial) of a change, which includes four phases: plan, do, study, and act. See the definition of "cycle" above. Sometimes known as plan, do, check, act (PDCA).

Process Change: A specific change in a process in the organization. More focused and detailed than a change concept, a process change describes what specific changes should occur. "Institute a pain management protocol for patients with moderate to severe pain" is an example of a process change.

Rapid Response Team: Rapid Response Teams include an intensive care unit doctor on duty plus an intensive care nurse who respond to calls from nurses on other floors to assess the condition of a patient.

Slots (also called discharge appointment times):   Defined appointment times available for scheduling discharges. For instance, discharge appointment times may be scheduled at 10 a.m., noon, 2 p.m., etc.

Surgical flow: The movement of patients into and out of the preoperative setting.

Team: The group of individuals, usually from multiple disciplines, that drives and participates in the improvement process.

Team triage: An innovative approach to patient entry in the ED. The patient is seen in triage by a nurse and a clinician (often a physician) and a diagnostic and therapeutic work up is initiated. This greatly shortens the patient arrival to doctor time and can also eliminate the need for putting the patient into a room or gurney in back.

Test: A small-scale trial of a new approach or a new process. A test is designed to learn if the change results in improvement and to fine-tune the change to fit the organization and patients. Tests are carried out using one or more PDSA cycles.

Throughput: The volume of patients admitted and discharged from the hospital, generally measured as number of inpatient admissions.

Upstream: Units transferring patients from one care area to another are considered "upstream."

Variation: The ebb and flow of patients arriving throughout the day.

Whiteboard: A write-on/wipe-off board placed next to the patient bed that can be used to post discharge time for all caregivers, patients, and family members to see and plan for.

About the Authors

Kirk Jensen, M.D., M.B.A, FACEP, has spent over 20 years in emergency medicine management and clinical care. Board-certified in emergency medicine, he has been medical director for several emergency departments and is vice president of clinical operations for BestPractices Inc., a group offering services in emergency physician leadership, management, staffing, clinical care, and patient satisfaction. Dr. Jensen is a faculty member of the Institute for Healthcare Improvement (IHI) focusing on patient flow, quality improvement, and patient satisfaction both within the ED and within the hospital. He currently chairs two IHI communities; (1) Improving Flow Through Acute Care Settings, and (2) Operational and Clinical Improvement in the Emergency Department. In addition, Dr. Jensen served on the expert panel and site examination team for Urgent Matters, a Robert Wood Johnson Foundation initiative focusing on helping hospitals eliminate ED crowding and congestion as well as preserving the healthcare safety net. Dr. Jensen is a successful speaker and coach for EDs across the country. He has expertise in workflow redesign, staff satisfaction, patient safety and satisfaction, project management, and other topics related to patient flow and process improvement.

Dr. Jensen holds a bachelor's degree in biology from the University of Illinois (Champaign) and a medical degree from the

University of Illinois (Chicago). He completed a residency in emergency medicine at the University of Chicago and an MBA at the University of Tennessee.

Thom A. Mayer, M.D., is president and chief executive officer of BestPractices, Inc., a national resource in physician leadership and management, which has placed major emphasis on patient flow and customer service.

Dr. Mayer has been the keynote speaker at numerous healthcare leadership conferences and also serves as the medical director of the NFL Players Association. He is one of America's foremost experts on healthcare customer service, patient flow, trauma and emergency care, pediatric emergency care, and medical leadership. He has published over 60 articles and 60 book chapters and has edited 12 medical textbooks. With Dr. Robert Cates, he authored the book *Leadership for Great Customer Service: Satisfied Patients, Satisfied Employees* (Health Administration Press 2004).

On September 11, 2001, Dr. Mayer served as one of the command physicians for the Pentagon Rescue Operation, coordinating medical assets at the site. His physicians at BestPractices, Inc., were also the first to successfully diagnose and treat inhalational anthrax victims during the 2001 anthrax crisis. Dr. Mayer is the lead editor of *Emergency Department Management: Principles and Applications*, the benchmark text on emergency leadership, and has served the Department of Defense and the Department of Homeland Security on Defense Science Board task forces on bioterrorism, homeland security, and consequences of weapons of mass destruction.

Shari J. Welch, M.D., FACEP, has been a practicing emergency physician for 20 years and a quality improvement consultant for 10 years. Dr. Welch trained in emergency medicine at Emory University, where she was chief resident, and she has served on the clinical faculty at Case Western Reserve University, Albany Medical College, and the University of Utah School of Medicine. Dr. Welch has worked as a consultant and educator in the area of quality improvement for Utah Emergency Physicians, Intermountain Health Care, The Schumacher Group, Emergency Services Partners, and Vanderbilt University. She has been a guest speaker at the Urgent Matters Conference, the ED Benchmarks Conference, the EDPMA Solutions Summit, VHA regional meetings, the AHRQ's national meeting, and American College of Emergency Physicians (ACEP) national meetings. Her quality improvement research has been published in numerous journals, including the *Annals of Emergency Medicine*, the *Journal of Emergency Medicine, Academic Emergency Medicine*, and *The Journal of Healthcare Quality*. Her work appears on the Six Sigma healthcare website and is featured on the Urgent Matters Robert Wood Johnson Foundation website. Currently Dr. Welch writes a regular column in *Emergency Medicine News* (which has a circulation of 40,000) titled "Quality Matters." Dr. Welch has worked with physicians and nurse managers in small, rural emergency departments with little information technology as well as large urban center emergency departments with advanced IT. She is currently a faculty member at the Institute for Healthcare Improvement and on the clinical faculty at the Urgent Matters Project for their Patient Flow Network. She has pioneered work on the "ED Dashboard Indicators," "Real Time Process Improvement," and "ED Reliability Models" concepts for emergency medicine at Intermountain Health Care.

Carol Haraden, Ph.D., is vice president at the Institute for Healthcare Improvement, where she is a member of the team responsible for developing innovative designs in patient care. She currently leads the Safer Patient's Initiative, a four-year project to improve patient safety in the United Kingdom sponsored by The Health Foundation. She has been a dean in higher education, a clinician, consultant, and researcher. Dr. Haraden has published several papers on measuring patient harm, improving intensive care outcomes, and innovation in heathcare design. She recently served on the Institute of Medicine Committee, Engineering Approaches to Improve Health Care. She is a judge for several national quality awards including the Quest for Quality Award sponsored by the AHA and the John Eisenberg Award for Patient Safety and Quality sponsored by the JCAHO. Dr. Haraden has served on AHRQ study sections and is a member of the JCAHO Sentinel Event Advisory Committee. She is an associate editor for the journal *Quality and Safety in Health Care*.

ABOUT IHI

Since its founding in 1991, the Institute for Healthcare Improvement (IHI) has been committed to helping grow and sustain a movement that is unifying our industry around the cause of improving health care for all. Our work for the past twelve years has focused on building the will and capacity for change in an industry in desperate need of innovation and redesign. Using this foundation, the IHI facilitates rich collaborative improvement work, identifying and spreading best practices, and achieving breakthrough results around the country and the globe. This work promotes and supports health care innovation, and ultimately seeks total system redesign. The IHI is recognized as a leader in creating change and driving health care improvement, nationally and internationally.